PRESS HERE!

SENSUAL MASSAGE
~ FOR BEGINNERS ~

PRESS HERE!

SENSUAL MASSAGE
~ FOR BEGINNERS ~

YOUR GUIDE TO PLEASURE AND INTIMACY

SYDNEY PRICE

Illustrations by
Emily Portnoi

FAIR WINDS

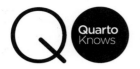

Inspiring | Educating | Creating | Entertaining

Brimming with creative inspiration, how-to projects, and useful information to enrich your everyday life, Quarto Knows is a favorite destination for those pursuing their interests and passions. Visit our site and dig deeper with our books into your area of interest: Quarto Creates, Quarto Cooks, Quarto Homes, Quarto Lives, Quarto Drives, Quarto Explores, Quarto Gifts, or Quarto Kids.

First Published in 2021 by Fair Winds Press,
an imprint of The Quarto Group.
100 Cummings Center, Suite 265-D,
Beverly, MA 01915, USA.
T (978) 282-9590 F (978) 283-2742

Fair Winds Press titles are also available at discount for retail, wholesale, promotional, and bulk purchase. For details, contact the Special Sales Manager by email at specialsales@quarto.com or by mail at The Quarto Group, Attn: Special Sales Manager, 100 Cummings Center, Suite 265-D, Beverly, MA 01915, USA.

25 24 23 22 21 1 2 3 4 5

ISBN: 978-1-58923-999-9

Digital edition published in 2021

QUAR.341499

Conceived, edited, and designed by Quarto Publishing plc.
6 Blundell Street, London N7 9BH

Editor: Claire Waite Brown
Designer and Illustrator: Emily Portnoi
Art Director: Gemma Wilson
Publisher: Samantha Warrington

Printed in Singapore

With the prevalence of sexually transmitted diseases, if you do not practice safe sex you are risking your life and your partner's life.

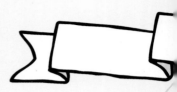

contents

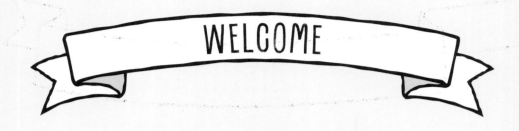

WELCOME

I'M SO GLAD YOU'RE HERE. CHOOSING TO LEARN ABOUT SENSUAL MASSAGE TAKES COURAGE, BUT IT'S WORTH IT. I WOULD KNOW; IT TOOK TIME FOR ME TO GATHER ENOUGH TO CHOOSE THIS PATH AS PART OF MY MASSAGE PROFESSION. I'M HAPPY I DID! IN MY TWENTIES, I HIT A WALL IN BOTH MY PERSONAL AND PROFESSIONAL LIVES. I REALIZED, WITH GRIEF AND CONFUSION, THAT I LIVED INSIDE AN INCREASINGLY NUMB BODY AND MY INTIMATE RELATIONSHIPS CONSISTENTLY LEFT ME DISSATISFIED. I BEGAN TO LEARN THAT MANY OF MY MASSAGE CLIENTS FELT THE SAME, BUT I HAD NO IDEA HOW TO HELP THEM WHEN I BARELY KNEW HOW TO HELP MYSELF. I SEARCHED FOR AND TRIED ANYTHING THAT MIGHT HELP ME FEEL AGAIN; MY BODY, MY PASSION, MY BOUNDARIES, MY SELF. LUCKILY, I STUMBLED UPON THE WORLD OF SENSUAL PRACTICE, INCLUDING SEXOLOGICAL BODYWORK AND SENSUAL MASSAGE.

I AM TRULY GRATEFUL. LEARNING TO GIVE AND RECEIVE PHYSICAL PLEASURE THROUGH TOUCH HAS OPENED MY HEART AND MIND IN UNEXPECTED WAYS. I KNOW AND TRUST MY BODY MORE, I COMMUNICATE WITH PARTNERS BETTER, AND I RECOGNIZE

HOW ESSENTIAL SENSUALITY IS TO MY OVERALL HEALTH. I TAKE RESPONSIBILITY FOR THE DESIRES THAT I CONSCIOUSLY EXPLORE, AND I UNDERSTAND BOUNDARIES, MY OWN AND THOSE OF OTHERS, WITH REFRESHING CLARITY. I DECIDED TO BECOME A CERTIFIED SEXOLOGICAL BODYWORKER, AND HELPING OTHERS EXPERIENCE THE MANY BENEFITS OF SENSUAL MASSAGE BRINGS ME JOY IN EVERY SESSION.

I BECAME A PROFESSIONAL, BUT YOU DON'T HAVE TO! SENSUAL MASSAGE IS EASY AND FUN TO LEARN. THIS BOOK WILL GIVE YOU THE TOOLS YOU NEED TO CREATE A PLEASURABLE EXPERIENCE, WHETHER YOU'RE SOLO OR PARTNERED. AFTER LEARNING THE FOUNDATIONS OF EMBODIED CONSENT, TUNING INTO PLEASURE, LOOKING AT SENSUAL ANATOMY, BUILDING YOUR SENSUAL TOOLBOX, AND FOLLOWING THE STEP-BY-STEP GUIDE, YOU'LL BE PRACTICING IN NO TIME!

GO FORWARD WITH AN OPEN MIND, STAY CURIOUS, AND YOU'LL FIND A WHOLE NEW WORLD OF POSSIBILITIES WAITING FOR YOU.

Sydney Price

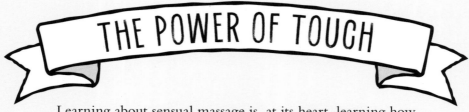

THE POWER OF TOUCH

Learning about sensual massage is, at its heart, learning how to touch. In both giving and receiving touch, what is really happening to our bodies, hearts, and minds?

How do we bring compassion and playfulness to the ways we touch one another? How do we track our sensations and see them as markers on the path to a greater understanding of ourselves and others? How do we do this with presence?

These are the kinds of questions that I believe sensual massage begins to answer, through all of our senses, but our sense of touch in particular. Our skin is our largest organ of perception and it is our clearest, most tangible boundary. Touch your own, and you feel an unmistakable, essential part of yourself. Touch another's, and you have access to a part of their unmistakable and essential self. Exchanging sensual touch can teach us how to take better care of one another. We can create a space where it is safe to explore our senses, desires, and boundaries, and to see where our explorations take us. Where else in our lives does such a space exist? We have the key right at our fingertips.

Reconnecting

Sensation is the language of the present moment. We live inside bodies that are designed to experience it in myriad ways. Our five senses are pathways that we can explore at length and incorporate into a sensual massage to deepen and enhance it. I include sexual anatomy in this perspective and write about it extensively in this book. Sadly, it is possible to live out our lives without ever accessing the potential pleasure of our sexual anatomy due to a lack of meaningful education and cultural taboos. Sensual massage can reconnect us to the lost parts of our bodies, remembering us to ourselves in profoundly beneficial ways.

Personal discovery

Learning to touch with curiosity, integrity, playfulness, and compassion can lead to surprising revelations, for yourself and for a partner. You may already be a step ahead of most people in knowing that the whole body, from your head to your toes, has the potential for pleasure. I've met people who can orgasm just from stimulating their ears or hands, or who regularly have orgasmic dreams! The possibilities are endless. If we approach a sensual massage practice as an opportunity to expand our access to sensations, including bliss and pleasure, we can cultivate a range of experiences, from the grounding to the elating and everything in between.

I hope this book serves as a blueprint for your own unique and special adventures. I hope that you discover things about yourself and your partners that surprise and delight you. Above all, I hope you find out for yourself what it means to touch and be touched.

ABOUT THE BOOK

The first two chapters use games and exercises to discover, communicate, and negotiate boundaries around touch, and ways to explore desires and practice sharing them.

Chapter 3 looks at pleasure anatomy, providing a deeper understanding of where and how your touch can be wonderfully pleasurable, and why, while in Chapter 4 you will learn how sights, sounds, scents, and touch come together to enhance your sensual massage experience.

The fifth chapter puts together the tools of the first four chapters and guides you through a complete, partnered massage sequence, including suggestions for how to open and close the practice and the importance of sharing after the session, while Chapter 6 considers the benefits of self-massage and ways to explore your self-pleasure experiences.

SPECIAL CONSIDERATIONS

There are many benefits to sensual massage, and I hope
you try it as often as you can! However, there are a few
instances in which it would be wise to abstain or make
some changes in order to practice safely.

Massage in pregnancy

In general, massage is a wonderful treatment
for a pregnant person, and after giving birth.
It helps with circulation, swelling joints, back
pain, and fatigue, to name just a few benefits.
Finding moments of sensuality can be helpful
during a time when so many significant
physical changes are taking place.

There are, however, a few considerations to
take into account when you're a pregnant
person receiving massage or working with a
pregnant partner.

RECEIVING SENSUAL MASSAGE WHILE PREGNANT

- Before receiving sensual massage during
  pregnancy, check with your physician about
  any possible contraindications. While it is
  rare, some individuals develop changes
  during pregnancy that increase their risk
  of blood clots, blood pressure changes, and
  other cardiovascular conditions that
  contraindicate massage.

- If you're cleared to receive a massage,
  fantastic! As your belly grows, try massage
  in a side-lying position with a pillow under
  your head and between your knees, along
  with any other props that make you most
  comfortable. A large wedge pillow can be
  used to assist with sitting up in a semi-
  reclined position, if you prefer.

- Don't lie for too long on your left side—
  stick to 20–30 minutes maximum. If you
  feel any lightheadedness before then, switch
  to your right side. The aorta, a major blood
  vessel, lies in the left side of your torso and
  can be compressed by the enlarged uterus if
  you lie on your left side for too long.

- Perineum massage is a great idea during
  pregnancy, both solo and with a partner.
  The perineum has to stretch during birth to
  accommodate the passage of the baby, and
  massage helps the tissue become more
  flexible and resilient.

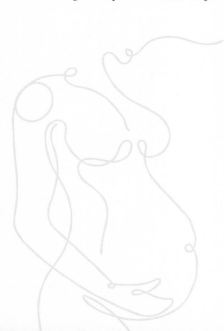

- If you're interested in receiving internal pelvic massage during pregnancy, consult with your physician about the safest way to proceed.

GIVING MASSAGE TO A PREGNANT PARTNER

- Before giving sensual massage to a pregnant partner, remember that the hormones involved in pregnancy make the joints extra flexible. Take care when trying any stretching or deep work around the joints.

- If your partner wants their belly massaged, move your strokes in the direction of digestion—up the right side, moving right to left under the ribs, down the left side, and left to right above the pubic bone.

- Avoid hard impact on the sacrum, the triangular bone at the base of the spine. A ligament stretches from this bone to the uterus, helping to keep it stable in the abdominal cavity. Gentle massage over the sacrum is fine.

- Some essential oils are better used during pregnancy than others; consult with an aromatherapy practitioner or guidebook before using essential oils. Check whether your partner has become extra sensitive to scents and would prefer to use an unscented massage oil.

Massage in the postpartum time

Increasing circulation, lymphatic drainage, warmth, and relaxation are very beneficial after giving birth. Receiving care in the midst of giving so much care to a newborn is crucial. Massage also provides a low-pressure, easeful way for partners to reconnect physically after the birth.

Here are a few considerations to remember for sensual massage during the postpartum time:

RECEIVING SENSUAL MASSAGE POSTPARTUM

- If you've had a cesarean section, wait six weeks before receiving any massage on your belly. Use warm castor oil on the scar; over time this will help the scar tissue to soften and become more flexible.

- As with during pregnancy, go gently when working around the joints since they will be more flexible due to hormonal changes.

- For at least 40 days after the birth use light pressure with strokes moving toward the heart. You and your partner may be tempted to use deeper pressure, and it won't cause any harm to apply a little more on the upper trapezius muscles or arms, but in general the lighter pressure will go farther in decreasing water retention, increasing lymphatic and blood circulation, aiding in the elimination of excess hormones, and much more.

- If you or your postpartum partner wants internal work, be sure any tears have had at least six weeks to heal and use warm castor oil. If there has been no tearing, I recommend still waiting at least 40 days until attempting internal work. Concentrate on moving slowly, noticing sensations and emotions as they arrive and practicing compassion for whatever they are. Your mindful, caring presence will be more helpful than an agenda to "fix" something. You may want to consult a pelvic-floor physical therapist or certified sexological bodyworker with regards to how best to work internally.

Contraindations for massage

Though it's unlikely you will come across
them, there are conditions that would be
negatively impacted by massage. If any of these
conditions apply to you or your partner, it's
best to check with a physician before trying
to practice massage.

- Fever

- Acute skin infections

- Cardiovascular conditions such as high
  blood pressure or an increased risk of
  blood clots

- Excessive consumption of alcohol

- If doing genital work, an active genital
  infection such as herpes sores, bacterial
  vaginosis, chlamydia, etc.

Safe sex

Of course, if you're sharing sensual massage
with a lover it might lead to some different
sensual activities, sexual intercourse being one
of many. To keep yourself and your partner
safe, take into account these considerations.

- If you are currently trying to avoid
  pregnancy and want to protect yourself
  and your partner from STIs, condoms are
  an excellent and reliable choice for safe
  penis–in–vagina intercourse.

- Use dental dams and condoms for
  safer oral sex.

- Use disposable gloves for genital touch if
  you have any cuts or scrapes on your hands
  or want to try anal touch.

- If using toys, don't share them among
  different partners and thoroughly clean them
  with toy-safe soap after use.

I AM NEVER MORE COURAGEOUS THAN WHEN
I AM EMBRACING IMPERFECTION, EMBRACING
VULNERABILITY, AND SETTING BOUNDARIES
WITH THE PEOPLE IN MY LIFE.

Brené Brown

CHAPTER 1

BOUNDARIES AND CONSENT

Beginning a book about sensual massage with a chapter on boundaries and consent might seem surprising, but trust me on this; when you start to embody your genuine "yes"s and "no"s, your pleasure in giving and receiving sensual touch can expand to surprising new heights.

The playful games I have detailed in this chapter will help you get in touch with and talk about your boundaries, and start building consent in an active and fun way.

WHY WE NEED BOUNDARIES AND CONSENT

The importance of establishing your "yes" and "no" comes down to your body and mind's perception of safety. So, how do we help ourselves and others feel safer? Enter boundaries and consent.

Humans are unconsciously hardwired to scan their environment for cues of safety and danger, all day long. This comes from our ancient roots, bygone eras spent running away from lions, tigers, and bears—oh my!—in prehistoric forests. Needless to say, most of us aren't running away from large animals these days. Instead, the chronic stress from our increasingly busy lives, attention-grabbing technology, jobs, and responsibilities, etc., has become the modern version of our ancient predators. Our brains are still doing their job to guard us from these less-tangible threats, and we rarely have a chance to fully relax. Using practices that show our minds and bodies we are safe can help us settle down in a world which is all keyed-up.

Establishing parameters

Boundaries and consent are often treated as intellectual concepts, static words that we may apply in our day-to-day lives only occasionally. Embodied consent—the practice of feeling boundaries on a physical level—turns our boundaries from ideas into a lived experience that can help us navigate our lives and relationships. It's taking the implicit and bringing it into the explicit, where we can become aware of and communicate our limits and what feels right for us in the moment. The communication of this information, and the agreements that follow between ourselves and our partners, is how we start to build a real experience of consent.

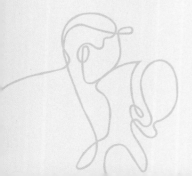

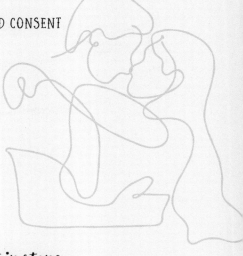

Think of consent as the container you create and step into when you start your massage adventure: once inside, you don't have to guess about the parameters and the limits, you don't have to worry so much about overstepping some line you can't see. Once you've done the work to establish those parameters you can start to play within them!

Not set in stone

It's important to note that the creation of this container of consent is ongoing. It's not a one-time event that stands written in stone forevermore (or until the massage ends). If the giver or receiver agreed to something at the onset, then later different sensations arise that tell them, "Hmm, no, actually, I'd rather not" or "Ooh, what about this instead?" they can pause, communicate, and then create a new and even better container. This ability to track present-moment feelings and sensations and communicate about them is incredibly valuable. That's why embodied consent is so useful in any touch exchange; when you are aware of your boundaries and share them, you're much more likely to get what you really want! I, for one, am all in favor of more people getting more of what they really want.

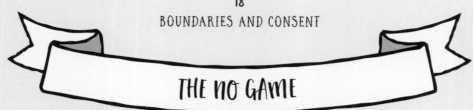

THE NO GAME

Practicing your "no" is a great way to empower your "yes," So, let's play the No Game.

Let's face it, no one really likes to hear "no," do they? Furthermore, how many of us feel comfortable saying it? This game, for both the one saying and the one hearing "no," provides great practice for diffusing this word of its negative charge.

At the end of the day, "no" is a gift; you are telling someone more about what you need and want in the moment, or someone else is giving you that vital information. Once equipped with this honest "no," an honest "yes" may be easier to find, and a sense of respect and clarity can grow in all of your massage practices.

Sitting together

If facing your partner is too challenging or makes you feel vulnerable, try sitting side by side with your shoulders touching, or sitting side by side facing opposite directions with your arms or legs touching.

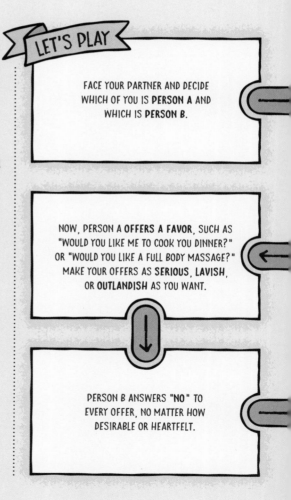

LET'S PLAY

FACE YOUR PARTNER AND DECIDE WHICH OF YOU IS **PERSON A** AND WHICH IS **PERSON B**.

NOW, PERSON A **OFFERS A FAVOR**, SUCH AS "WOULD YOU LIKE ME TO COOK YOU DINNER?" OR "WOULD YOU LIKE A FULL BODY MASSAGE?" MAKE YOUR OFFERS AS **SERIOUS**, **LAVISH**, OR **OUTLANDISH** AS YOU WANT.

PERSON B ANSWERS **"NO"** TO EVERY OFFER, NO MATTER HOW DESIRABLE OR HEARTFELT.

PERSON A **ASKS** PERSON B FOR A **FAVOR**, SUCH AS "WILL YOU DO MY DISHES?" OR "WILL YOU COME BY AND WALK MY DOG?" GET CREATIVE, YOU CAN MAKE YOUR REQUESTS AS **SERIOUS** OR **SILLY** AS YOU LIKE.

PERSON B ANSWERS **"NO"** TO EVERY SINGLE REQUEST. NO MATTER HOW MUCH YOU WANT TO SAY "YES," PRACTICE SAYING **"NO."**

PAUSE. CHECK IN WITH YOUR BODY; HOW DOES IT FEEL TO HEAR "NO" AND SAY "THANK YOU" AFTERWARD? HOW DOES IT FEEL TO SAY IT AND BE THANKED? **NOTICE ANY SENSATIONS** THIS MIGHT BRING UP FOR YOU.

PERSON A SAYS **"THANK YOU"** AFTER HEARING EACH "NO" FROM PERSON B. CONTINUE LIKE THIS FOR AT LEAST **THREE MINUTES.**

PERSON A SAYS **"THANK YOU,"** AFTER HEARING EACH "NO" FROM PERSON B. CONTINUE LIKE THIS FOR AT LEAST **THREE MINUTES.**

PAUSE AGAIN, CHECKING IN TO SEE HOW THIS ROUND MIGHT BRING UP DIFFERENT **SENSATIONS AND THOUGHTS** FOR EACH PERSON. AFTER PLAYING BOTH ROLES, **SHARE** WITH EACH OTHER: "HOW WAS THAT FOR YOU?"

THE YES, NO, MAYBE GAME

In the Yes, No, Maybe Game we start to introduce more possibilities. For now, the idea is just to notice the different experiences of expressing and hearing these answers, not following through on them.

"Maybe" is a particularly useful word; when we're not an "absolutley, yes!" but we're not a "no way!" either, "maybe" can step in and invite more communication and negotiation.

Pay attention

While it may sound strange (or clichéd) to think that your physical sensations are connected to your thoughts, becoming aware of this connection is a great way to start working on embodied consent; "yes," "no," or "maybe" can be intellectual, but they can also be physical experiences. Pay attention to your body and it can give you valuable clues as to where your boundaries lie and how you can navigate consent.

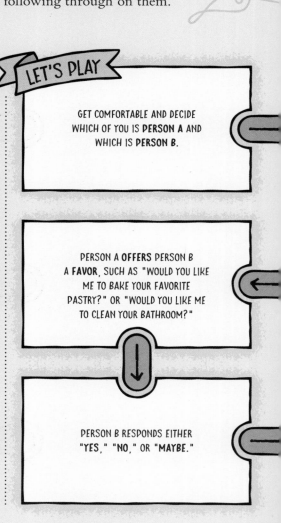

LET'S PLAY

GET COMFORTABLE AND DECIDE WHICH OF YOU IS **PERSON A** AND WHICH IS **PERSON B**.

PERSON A **OFFERS** PERSON B A **FAVOR**, SUCH AS "WOULD YOU LIKE ME TO BAKE YOUR FAVORITE PASTRY?" OR "WOULD YOU LIKE ME TO CLEAN YOUR BATHROOM?"

PERSON B RESPONDS EITHER "YES," "NO," OR "MAYBE."

THE YES, NO, MAYBE GAME

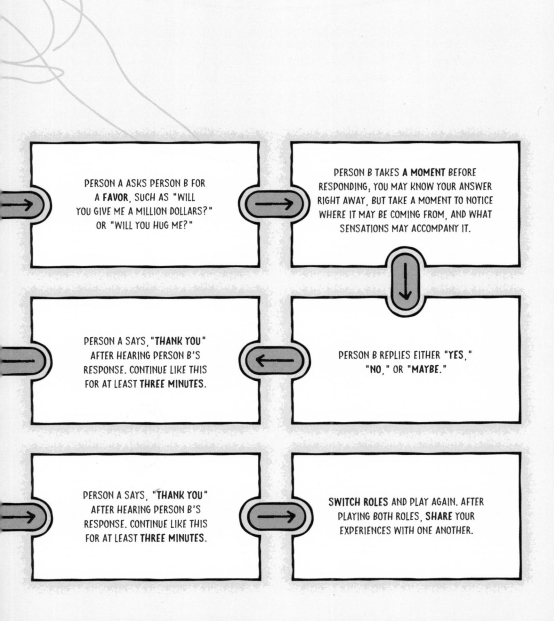

PERSON A ASKS PERSON B FOR A **FAVOR**, SUCH AS "WILL YOU GIVE ME A MILLION DOLLARS?" OR "WILL YOU HUG ME?"

PERSON B TAKES **A MOMENT** BEFORE RESPONDING, YOU MAY KNOW YOUR ANSWER RIGHT AWAY, BUT TAKE A MOMENT TO NOTICE WHERE IT MAY BE COMING FROM, AND WHAT SENSATIONS MAY ACCOMPANY IT.

PERSON A SAYS, **"THANK YOU"** AFTER HEARING PERSON B'S RESPONSE. CONTINUE LIKE THIS FOR AT LEAST **THREE MINUTES**.

PERSON B REPLIES EITHER **"YES,"** **"NO,"** OR **"MAYBE."**

PERSON A SAYS, **"THANK YOU"** AFTER HEARING PERSON B'S RESPONSE. CONTINUE LIKE THIS FOR AT LEAST **THREE MINUTES**.

SWITCH ROLES AND PLAY AGAIN. AFTER PLAYING BOTH ROLES, **SHARE** YOUR EXPERIENCES WITH ONE ANOTHER.

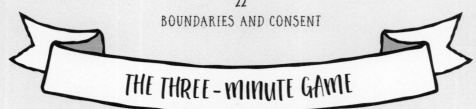

THE THREE-MINUTE GAME

Practicing setting boundaries before adding touch is important so that when we include more physical interaction we have a good foundation. Our ability to stay aware of our sensations and build trust with our partner is given another dimension when we add touch.

The Three-Minute Game, created by life coach Harry Faddis, is an excellent way of adding that dimension to your boundary experiment, since it can provide a very playful and lighthearted approach.

The game is built on two questions:
- How do you want to touch me for three minutes?
- How do you want me to touch you for three minutes?

Touch for pleasure

The question, "How do you want to touch me for three minutes?" gives the touching partner a unique opportunity to touch for their pleasure. This can be an edgy experience for many reasons, not least of which is our cultural relationship to taking pleasure for ourselves and how often this is considered selfish or taboo. But the chance to practice this kind of touch in a consensual way can teach us how to enjoy ourselves and others so much more! So, take a chance on taking some pleasure all for yourself and see what happens.

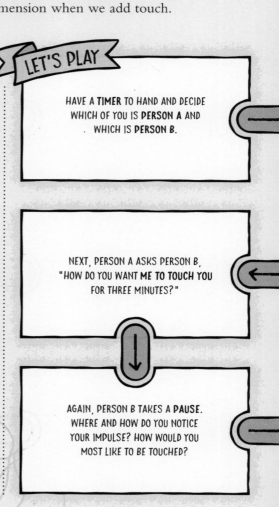

LET'S PLAY

HAVE A **TIMER** TO HAND AND DECIDE WHICH OF YOU IS **PERSON A** AND WHICH IS **PERSON B**.

NEXT, PERSON A ASKS PERSON B, "HOW DO YOU WANT **ME TO TOUCH YOU** FOR THREE MINUTES?"

AGAIN, PERSON B TAKES A **PAUSE**. WHERE AND HOW DO YOU NOTICE YOUR IMPULSE? HOW WOULD YOU MOST LIKE TO BE TOUCHED?

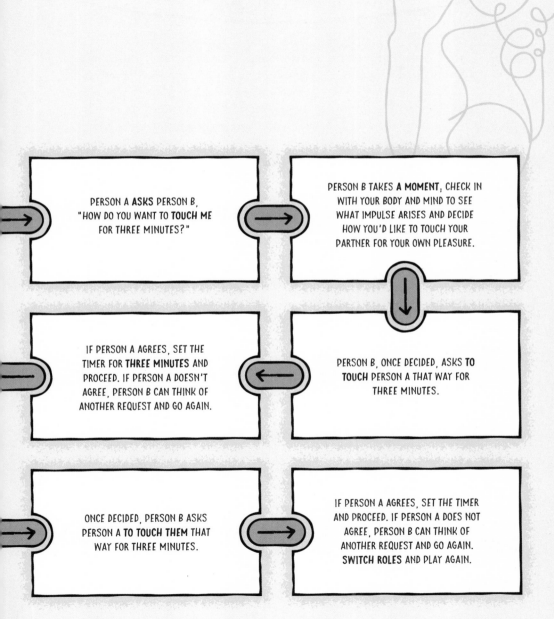

PERSON A **ASKS** PERSON B, "HOW DO YOU WANT TO **TOUCH ME** FOR THREE MINUTES?"

PERSON B TAKES **A MOMENT**; CHECK IN WITH YOUR BODY AND MIND TO SEE WHAT IMPULSE ARISES AND DECIDE HOW YOU'D LIKE TO TOUCH YOUR PARTNER FOR YOUR OWN PLEASURE.

IF PERSON A AGREES, SET THE TIMER FOR **THREE MINUTES** AND PROCEED. IF PERSON A DOESN'T AGREE, PERSON B CAN THINK OF ANOTHER REQUEST AND GO AGAIN.

PERSON B, ONCE DECIDED, ASKS **TO TOUCH** PERSON A THAT WAY FOR THREE MINUTES.

ONCE DECIDED, PERSON B ASKS PERSON A **TO TOUCH THEM** THAT WAY FOR THREE MINUTES.

IF PERSON A AGREES, SET THE TIMER AND PROCEED. IF PERSON A DOES NOT AGREE, PERSON B CAN THINK OF ANOTHER REQUEST AND GO AGAIN. **SWITCH ROLES** AND PLAY AGAIN.

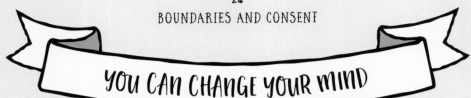

YOU CAN CHANGE YOUR MIND

After you've agreed to do something, you can change your mind.
After you've declined to do something, you can change your mind. In
the middle of experiencing something you don't genuinely enjoy, you
can change your mind. In the middle of experiencing exactly what
you asked for, you can change your mind.

Changing your mind can look like asking for a slight adjustment, or something completely different. Changing your mind can look like taking a moment to pause and check in with your body. Changing your mind can look like coming to a full stop and leaving the game, massage, etc., for another day. It looks like taking care of yourself, and, by proxy, your partner and anyone else you are playing with. It doesn't make you high maintenance, needy, confused, or any other ridiculous assumption some (or we, ourselves) might make when you change your mind in order to create an experience that genuinely reflects what you desire in the moment.

Having the capacity to listen to your body, know your boundaries, and change your mind when or if you need to means you are in charge. You are in the driver's seat of this experience, not the passenger's seat! Please, do not simply tolerate anything. Instead, find out how to enjoy everything by listening well to yourself and changing your mind, whenever you want to!

HELPFUL QUESTIONS

These questions may help you to understand and vocalize your experiences of the games in this chapter.

WHERE AND HOW DO YOU FEEL YOUR "YES," "NO," AND "MAYBE"? TRY USING SENSATION LANGUAGE SUCH AS TINGLING, WARMTH, CONSTRICTION, ETC., AND SPECIFIC LOCATIONS IN THE BODY.

. . . .

IS IT EASY OR CHALLENGING TO SAY "NO"? TO SAY "YES"?

. . . .

HOW DO YOU KNOW WHEN YOU'RE RECEIVING EXACTLY WHAT YOU ASKED FOR? WHAT DOES THAT FEEL LIKE IN YOUR BODY? AGAIN, AIM FOR SPECIFIC SENSATIONS AND LOCATIONS, FOR EXAMPLE "I FEEL A FLUTTERING IN MY BELLY' OR "THERE ARE CHAMPAGNE BUBBLES BEHIND MY RIBS."

. . . .

HOW DO YOU KNOW WHEN YOU WANT TO CHANGE YOUR MIND?

. . . .

WHAT IS IT LIKE TO TOUCH YOUR PARTNER FOR YOUR OWN PLEASURE? HOW IS IT DIFFERENT THAN TOUCHING THEM FOR THEIR PLEASURE?

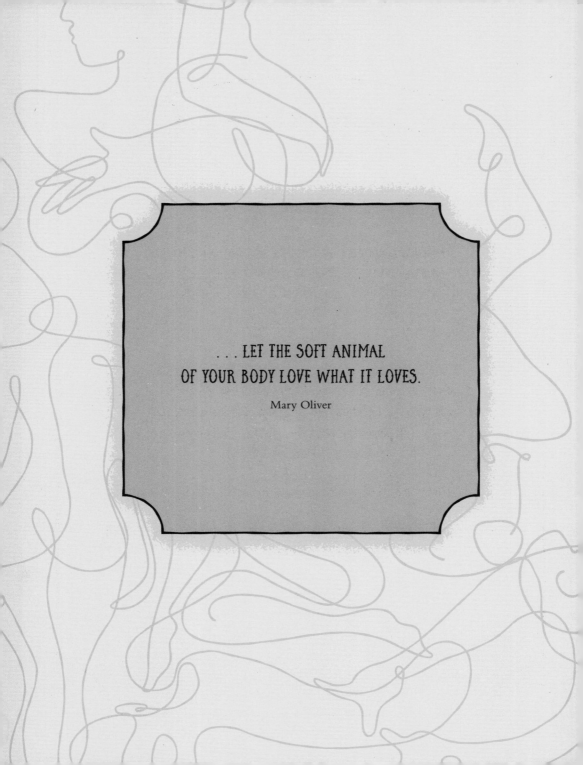

. . . LET THE SOFT ANIMAL
OF YOUR BODY LOVE WHAT IT LOVES.

Mary Oliver

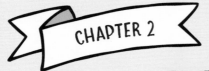

CHAPTER 2

THE PATH TO PLEASURE

This chapter is all about finding pleasure and orienting to it.

Since the early days of wandering through the wilderness or running from predators, the human brain has scanned its environment for threat. This has created a nifty little survival mechanism called the negativity bias. Just like it sounds, we are biased toward negativity in order to remember which primordial plants and animals to avoid. In the modern world this can translate to a frustrating inability to become aware of and focus on sensations of pleasure.

The good news is we have bodies and minds that are remarkably adaptable! Once given the tools and practices to notice, orient to, and concentrate on pleasure, we can increase our capacity to feel it tenfold. Learning how to strengthen that receptivity and strike a better balance between your survival wiring and your pleasure capacity can set your massage experience, and any intimate sharing, up for success.

START WITH YOUR HANDS

There are 17,000 touch receptors in the palm of your hand. 17,000! Since you've got two hands . . . well, someone else can do the math, but that's quite a lot combined. Let's explore all of that sensitivity and learn about how to take pleasure from touching.

"Taking" gets a bad rap in most societies. No one wants to be selfish or accused of taking too much of any one thing: space, time, resources, or even something as wonderful as pleasure. But it is our ability to take in sensations from our hands, and our whole bodies, that holds the key to turning a massage from a one-way street all about giving, to a two-way, collaborative exchange that is mutually beneficial, exploratory, and pleasurable.

Relaxing or arousing

Eventually, you may be surprised to find this exercise relaxing or even arousing. You're tapping into your innate pleasure muscles, which do wonders to help us lower our stress levels and increase our arousal.

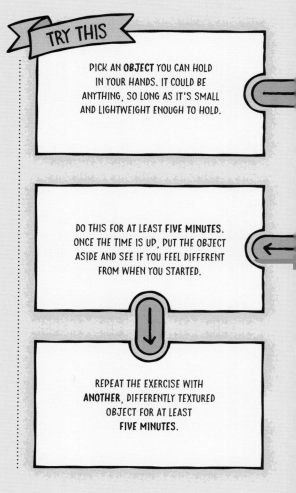

TRY THIS

PICK AN **OBJECT** YOU CAN HOLD IN YOUR HANDS. IT COULD BE ANYTHING, SO LONG AS IT'S SMALL AND LIGHTWEIGHT ENOUGH TO HOLD.

DO THIS FOR AT LEAST **FIVE MINUTES**. ONCE THE TIME IS UP, PUT THE OBJECT ASIDE AND SEE IF YOU FEEL DIFFERENT FROM WHEN YOU STARTED.

REPEAT THE EXERCISE WITH **ANOTHER**, DIFFERENTLY TEXTURED OBJECT FOR AT LEAST **FIVE MINUTES**.

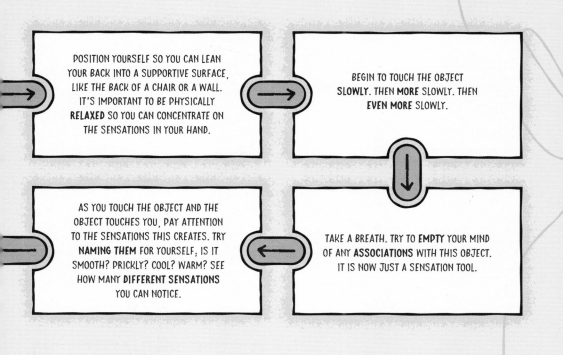

POSITION YOURSELF SO YOU CAN LEAN YOUR BACK INTO A SUPPORTIVE SURFACE, LIKE THE BACK OF A CHAIR OR A WALL. IT'S IMPORTANT TO BE PHYSICALLY **RELAXED** SO YOU CAN CONCENTRATE ON THE SENSATIONS IN YOUR HAND.

BEGIN TO TOUCH THE OBJECT **SLOWLY**. THEN **MORE** SLOWLY. THEN **EVEN MORE** SLOWLY.

AS YOU TOUCH THE OBJECT AND THE OBJECT TOUCHES YOU, PAY ATTENTION TO THE SENSATIONS THIS CREATES. TRY **NAMING THEM** FOR YOURSELF: IS IT SMOOTH? PRICKLY? COOL? WARM? SEE HOW MANY **DIFFERENT SENSATIONS** YOU CAN NOTICE.

TAKE A BREATH. TRY TO **EMPTY** YOUR MIND OF ANY **ASSOCIATIONS** WITH THIS OBJECT. IT IS NOW JUST A SENSATION TOOL.

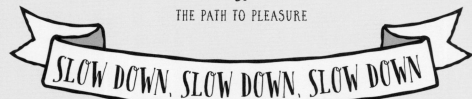

SLOW DOWN, SLOW DOWN, SLOW DOWN

Our minds move faster than our bodies. They whirl so fast, so continuously, that we can go through an entire day without noticing our bodies or the sensations they are experiencing. Slowing down is an antidote to this disconnection.

When we move at our body's pace, rather than our mind's pace, we have the opportunity to notice more sensation. Once we notice, we can follow; once following, we can learn new things, be surprised, delighted, and intrigued by what lies beneath our hands. Think of it as similar to meditation, but instead of emptying your mind you are trying to fill it with the information coming from your hands. It automatically places your awareness in the present, which is the only place our sensory receptors live.

Connected to the present

When you are giving and receiving a sensual massage, the practice of slowing down can help keep both you and your partner connected to the sensations happening in the present moment. The giver can follow the feeling under their hands and learn about their partner's body, along with enjoying the textures of their skin and the shape of their muscles and bones. The receiver can more deeply relax into the touch as a slow pace has a tonic effect on the nervous system and can help them stay grounded and present.

TRY THIS

GET COMFORTABLE WITH YOUR PARTNER AND DECIDE WHICH OF YOU IS **PERSON A** AND WHICH IS **PERSON B**.

DO THIS FOR AT LEAST **FIVE MINUTES**. WHEN THE TIME IS UP, **PAUSE** FOR A MOMENT TO INTEGRATE. **SHARE** HOW THAT FELT FOR EACH OF YOU.

SWITCH ROLES AND PLAY AGAIN.

SLOW DOWN, SLOW DOWN, SLOW DOWN

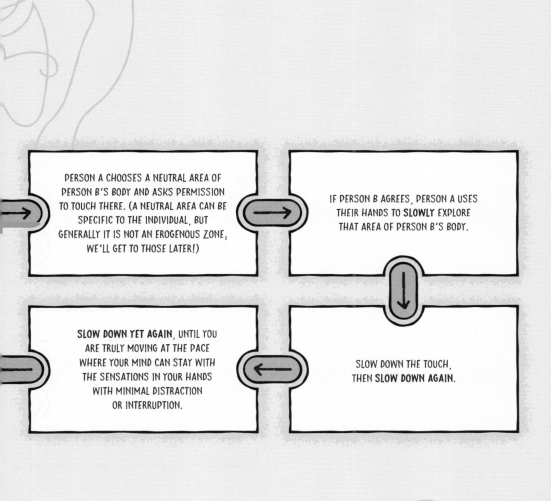

PERSON A CHOOSES A NEUTRAL AREA OF PERSON B'S BODY AND ASKS PERMISSION TO TOUCH THERE. (A NEUTRAL AREA CAN BE SPECIFIC TO THE INDIVIDUAL, BUT GENERALLY IT IS NOT AN EROGENOUS ZONE; WE'LL GET TO THOSE LATER!)

IF PERSON B AGREES, PERSON A USES THEIR HANDS TO **SLOWLY** EXPLORE THAT AREA OF PERSON B'S BODY.

SLOW DOWN YET AGAIN, UNTIL YOU ARE TRULY MOVING AT THE PACE WHERE YOUR MIND CAN STAY WITH THE SENSATIONS IN YOUR HANDS WITH MINIMAL DISTRACTION OR INTERRUPTION.

SLOW DOWN THE TOUCH, THEN **SLOW DOWN AGAIN**.

CREATING DIFFERENT SENSATIONS

Think of your body as one gigantic instrument—in many ways, it is exactly that! Every nerve receptor on your skin is a doorway for information to flow through, like a key on a piano that, once stuck, sends a signal vibrating through the body and up to your brain. There, it is processed and sent back out as your perceived thoughts and actions; your music.

When we take advantage of as many of these keys as possible to create new and novel sensations for ourselves, we can actively participate in this flow of information and what comes out of it. We make our own music; we are an instrument that can play itself. So, what would you like to play? Better yet, how would you like to play?

Sense of touch

Try this exercise to experiment with new sensations. Consider taking part while blindfolded, to enhance your sense of touch and help remove any associations you might have with the objects by sight. Over time, you can expand this exercise to include more and more of your body.

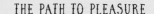

TRY THIS

GATHER A SMALL COLLECTION OF OBJECTS THAT ARE EASY TO HOLD AND MOVE IN YOUR HANDS. TRY TO CHOOSE A **VARIETY OF OBJECTS** WITH DIFFERENT TEXTURES, TEMPERATURES, AND WEIGHTS.

TRY THIS FOR AT LEAST **TEN MINUTES**, SWITCHING YOUR OBJECTS AND CREATING NEW SENSATIONS EVERY FEW MINUTES OR SO. AT THE END, TAKE A MOMENT TO **INTEGRATE** THE **EXPERIENCE** AND SEE IF YOU FEEL ANY DIFFERENT FROM WHEN YOU STARTED PLAYING.

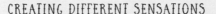

WITH ONE HAND, BEGIN **TOUCHING** YOUR OTHER HAND AND FOREARM WITH ONE OF **YOUR OBJECTS**. DISCOVER ALL THE DIFFERENT WAYS THIS OBJECT CAN CONTACT YOUR SKIN AND CREATE SENSATION: GET CREATIVE, EXPLORE, AND STAY PRESENT TO HOW YOU FEEL.

AFTER A FEW MINUTES, CHOOSE A DIFFERENT OBJECT FOR YOUR "GIVING" HAND TO TOUCH TO YOUR "RECEIVING" HAND. AFTER ANOTHER FEW MINUTES, **SWITCH AGAIN.**

IF YOU'RE PLAYING WITH AN OBJECT AND FEEL LOST OR RUN OUT OF IDEAS, JUST **PAUSE** FOR A MOMENT AND BREATHE. GIVE YOURSELF SPACE FOR A NEW IDEA TO ARISE. WHATEVER IT IS, FOLLOW IT WITH **CURIOSITY** AND SUSPEND YOUR JUDGMENT FOR AS LONG AS YOU CAN. WE'RE JUST IMPROVISING SOME NEW MUSIC, HERE!

ORIENT TO PLEASURE

All of the exercises in this chapter are designed to help you focus on sensation in a general sense, but what about pleasure, specifically? The more you can feel your body, the more likely you are to notice pleasurable sensations, but how can we stay with and expand that pleasure when we find it?

Think back to the exercises you've tried. Was there a sensation you found especially enjoyable? Return to that sensation, either giving it to yourself or receiving it from a partner. What happens in your body while you are experiencing this pleasure? Do you hold your breath or tense your muscles? Does your mind automatically wander somewhere else, or fill with concerns such as "Is this OK?" "Is this too much?" or "Too weird?" Do you get bored after five seconds? No judgment; just notice.

Breathe

Now, take a breath. When you find yourself pulling away from pleasure, take a breath and exhale slowly. Breathing is a great way to return to your senses and the present moment. It helps loosen tension in the body which can quite literally squeeze pleasure out of the picture. It creates a moment to slow down, drop in, and refocus. Let your breath help you find your way back to the pleasure.

Notice and breathe again

As you move throughout your day, try to notice any pleasure you come across. It could be simple like the feeling of warm water running over your hands while you do the dishes, or something more intense like a deep kiss from a lover. Whatever it is, remember to breathe when you find it. See if your breath can help you suspend the moment a little longer, relish the pleasure a little more. Tune your instrument to the things you enjoy. Make this a daily practice and your sensual massage experiences will benefit immensely.

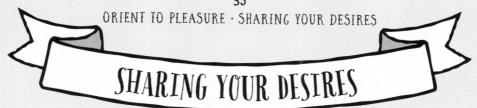

SHARING YOUR DESIRES

As you are exploring what you find pleasurable, my courageous
reader, you may wonder how to get from here to communicating
these discoveries with your partner. It can be a tongue-tying task,
one that requires vulnerability, trust, and letting go of any
attachment to the outcome.

Betty Martin, a fantastic sexuality educator and
creator of The School of Consent, breaks down
the journey to sharing a desire like this:

Each step acts like the piece of a bridge
between your awareness of a desire and your
physical experience of it. We've spent time in
this chapter working on staying present to our
sensations through exercises that put our minds
in our hands; slowing down; creating new
sensations; and breathing into our pleasure.
Accepting, trusting, and sharing are the next
steps to take.

Is one step easier than another? Do you find
yourself judging a desire, unable to accept it?
Or do you second-guess yourself, unable to
trust that feeling of "Yes, I do want that?"
Finally, at the last step, what words do you
turn to when you feel ready to share?

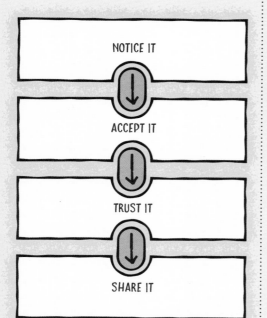

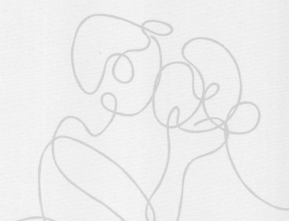

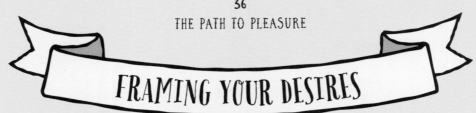

FRAMING YOUR DESIRES

Framing your desires is an opportunity for curious exploration, by which you can ease any performance pressure on you or your partner's part.

Remember the negotiation and communication skills from the Boundaries and Consent chapter? They can come in handy here too. Each time you want to explore a desire with a partner, practice walking the bridge discussed on page 35 and, eventually, it will become second nature to notice, accept, trust, and share it.

TRY THIS

Here are a few suggestions to try—feel free to improvise and play with these as much as you like:

"I REALLY LOVE THE FEELING OF _ _ _ _ _ _ _, I WANT TO TRY THAT WITH YOU."

"EARLIER, WHEN I DID _ _ _ _ _ _ _ _ WITH MY HANDS,
IT FELT REALLY COOL. COULD YOU TRY DOING THAT TO ME?"

"I GET EXCITED WHEN I THINK ABOUT DOING _ _ _ _ _ _ _ _ _ ."

"I'M NOT EXACTLY SURE HOW TO ASK FOR WHAT I WANT, BUT I THINK IT'S
LIKE _ _ _ _ _ _ _ _ _ AND/OR _ _ _ _ _ _ _, COULD WE TRY TO FIGURE IT OUT TOGETHER?"

HELPFUL QUESTIONS

Use these questions to help you to understand and communicate your experiences of the exercises in this chapter.

WHAT HELPS YOU FOCUS ON PLEASURE?

. . . .

WHAT TENDS TO DISTRACT YOU?

. . . .

WHAT HELPS YOU TUNE INTO A DESIRE?

. . . .

WHAT KINDS OF TOUCH AND SENSATIONS DID YOU
ESPECIALLY ENJOY CREATING FOR YOURSELF,
OR RECEIVING FROM A PARTNER?

. . . .

WHAT IS THE EASIEST WAY FOR YOU
TO COMMUNICATE A DESIRE?

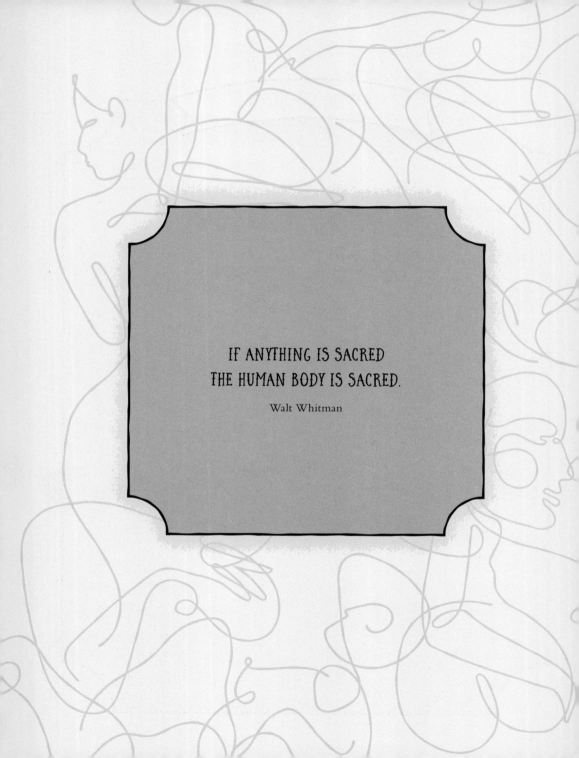

IF ANYTHING IS SACRED
THE HUMAN BODY IS SACRED.

Walt Whitman

CHAPTER 3

THE ANATOMY OF AROUSAL

Our standard sex education may give us some foundational tools—mainly how to avoid STIs and pregnancy—but it is seriously lacking in pleasure information. Let us now correct this oversight!

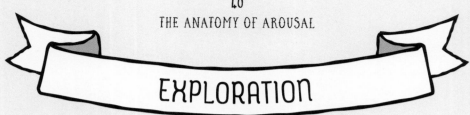

EXPLORATION

The more you know your pleasure anatomy, the more you can take advantage of it. With this knowledge, communication between yourself and a partner can be clearer and more specific; with more opportunities for getting what you really want!

The vulva

The vulva has been historically misrepresented and misunderstood. It enjoyed some acceptance in anatomical literature for a time; however, when the patriarchal, male-dominated field of early medicine realized the vulva had nothing to do with reproduction, they quickly removed it from textbooks and curricula. This deliberate oversight lasted for centuries. It is only fairly recently that anatomists, medical scientists, and everyday people are fully recognizing and appreciating this remarkable organ and all of its structures.

On pages 42–43 we will learn about the external vulval anatomy, and concentrate on the internal on pages 44–45, focusing on the areas that are usually underrepresented.

STAGED AROUSAL

The vulva becomes aroused in stages. On average, it takes 30–45 minutes for the entire vulva (external and internal structures) to become fully aroused. Arousal takes the form of engorgement of erectile tissues such as the clitoris, for one example. (Yes, female bodies get erections, too! The sexual organs of male and female bodies are made of the same tissue that develops in different ways en utero. Think about that!)

As you explore these parts of yourself, either solo or partnered, take some time to notice any changes in look and feel, and consider these signposts on your path to full arousal.

PHYSICAL EXPLORATION
Over the next few pages, I recommend following with your hands on your body as well as with your eyes on the page! For internal exploration, keep fingernails trimmed and use plenty of lubrication.

The penis

The external location of the penis makes it a little less mysterious then the vulva, but even so, there are anatomical landmarks and physiological events that are usually left out of penis arousal education. Once again, I'll highlight a few things most penis owners may not be familiar with, and leave out more well-known pleasure spots.

PRIORITIES

Given the prevalence of pornography, lack of somatic education, and prioritizing erection and orgasm over different experiences, many people find it challenging to change their habits of touch. Taking the time to slowly explore your penis without the agenda of getting an erection or having an orgasm can be very illuminating.

The anus

The anus is a sensitive organ of eroticism just as much as it is an organ of elimination. Its dual function has contributed in part to the taboo around exploring its sensual potential; many people are concerned about hygiene and safety and therefore stay away from exploring their anus. We'll cover how to enjoy this area safely and cleanly.

FURTHER RESOURCES

I have chosen to concentrate on the misunderstood and misrepresented areas of arousal anatomy, which means I may leave some obvious things out. Don't worry, as there are some excellent resources on page 128 that you can turn to for more in-depth study.

EXTERNAL VULVA ANATOMY

Areas of vulva anatomy are commonly overlooked, and here
I will focus on those areas that are usually underrepresented.

THE LIPS

The **outer** and **inner lips** (labia) of the vulva
are often overlooked as a source of sensual
pleasure. Try rolling the outer lips between
your fingers and stretching the inner lips,
playing with these remarkably flexible and
malleable tissues. Notice any interesting or
pleasurable sensations you find here. The inner
lips change quite noticeably over the course of
becoming aroused, darkening in color and
swelling outward. I believe this accounts for
the common comparison of the vulva to
flowers; it blooms!

THE URETHRAL OPENING

Part the inner lips and you'll see a smooth
surface, topped by the juncture of the lips and
bottomed by the entrance to the vagina, the
vaginal introitus. Between these two landmarks
is the **urethral opening**. It may be hard to
pinpoint, requiring a flashlight and hand
mirror. I like to include it because many vulva
owners are very surprised to discover this area
can hold a lot of pleasure for them. It also
"blooms" over the course of arousal, darkening
and puckering up.

THE INTROITUS

Underneath the urethral opening is the
opening to the vagina, or the **introitus**.
Another area that changes in color and tension
during arousal, it is rich in nerve endings and
can be missed in the rush to penetration. Press
experimentally into the muscle tissue around
the opening and you'll contact your pelvic
floor musculature. See if you can hug the
introitus up into your center and you'll be
contracting those muscles.

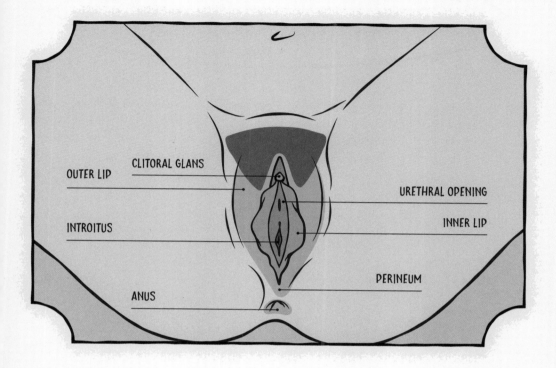

OUTER LIP

CLITORAL GLANS

INTROITUS

ANUS

URETHRAL OPENING

INNER LIP

PERINEUM

THE PERINEUM

Located between the vaginal introitus and the anus, the **perineum** plays an important role in overall pelvic and sexual health. It is the connective tissue linchpin of what's called your pelvic "floor," though it's more like a hammock of muscles and fascia that supports your internal organs. The perineal sponge is also located here, internally, a maze of blood vessels that engorges during arousal. Massaging here with some warm, skin-friendly oil can help the entire pelvic floor relax and soften—a necessary prerequisite for more circulation and sensation in the pelvis.

NATURAL CHANGES

Notice how many of these structures change in color, size, and tension over the course of becoming aroused. Consider touching yourself in front of a mirror, or ask a partner to report on visible changes in the vulva while you're playing. Recognizing the signs of arousal can help you traverse its path with more confidence.

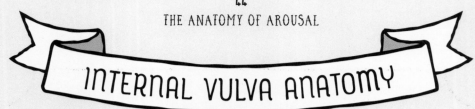

INTERNAL VULVA ANATOMY

You'll notice I use the word "cavern" rather than "canal" to describe the vagina, which is anatomically more accurate. The vagina is not an open tube but rather more like a voluminous pocket that can shape-shift to adapt to the contents inside. "Cave of Wonders" is also perfectly suitable.

If you are following along with your hands—and I hope you are!—lubrication would be excellent here.

THE VESTIBULAR BULBS

The **vestibular bulbs** are located fairly close to the entrance of the vagina, internally. Press a finger into the sidewalls of the vagina and slightly up, and you'll be in their vicinity. These bulbs gradually swell with blood and become erect, creating the "hugging" sensation inside the cavern. This swelling creates a pleasurable pressure on nearby internal pleasure anatomy. It also causes the external vulva to puff up and bloom outward. You can contact these bulbs by massaging down and into the outer labia of the vulva, and into the sidewalls inside the cavern.

CLITORAL SHAFT AND LEGS

The **clitoris** is an internal structure. Oh yes! While the **glans**, or head, of the clitoris understandably steals the show most often, the whole clitoris is actually a large organ that stretches far inside the body. It frames the vagina in a shape quite reminiscent of a wishbone. Find the hood of the clitoris, which is formed by the topmost juncture of the inner labia that covers and protects the glans. Gently press into it, moving your finger up toward your pubic bone and tummy. This is the **shaft** of the clitoris, containing many sensual nerves and sometimes passed over in favor of the electric sensations in the glans. Back inside the vaginal cavern, the **legs** of the clitoris mirror the position and direction of the vestibular bulbs on either side. The glans, shaft, and legs of the clitoris all increase in size and become erect during the stages of arousal, once again contributing to increased sensation, pleasurable pressure, and the outward blooming of the whole vulva.

The nerve endings inside the vaginal cavern respond to pressure, not touch. With that in mind, some anatomists believe the sensations of pleasure inside come more from the legs of the clitoris than from the walls themselves.

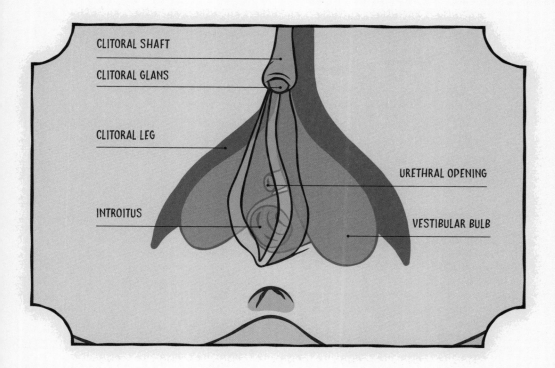

CLITORAL SHAFT

CLITORAL GLANS

CLITORAL LEG

INTROITUS

URETHRAL OPENING

VESTIBULAR BULB

THE G-SPOT

Many are familiar with the G-spot, since it's been exhaustively covered in almost every magazine marketed toward women since the dawn of print media's obsession with sex advice. That said, when have you heard it referred to as a crest, and not just a spot? It has also been recently renamed by Australian anatomist and urologist Dr Helen O'Connell as the "CUV"—Clitoral Urethral Vaginal—complex, recognizing the urethral sponge's role in contributing to the sensitivity of this area.

The CUV/G-crest is an area of erectile tissue located just behind the upper wall of the vagina, facing the belly. It surrounds the urethra all the way up to the bladder, thereby becoming a crest or area rather than a "spot," and where exactly it feels sensitive differs from person to person. As it expands and becomes erect it grows more and more sensitive. In some vulva owners, it can trigger ejaculation when stimulated in high arousal. Unaroused, it can be relatively lacking in sensation or even be unpleasant to touch, so tread gently if you are not currently aroused. It is typically described as having a different texture than the rest of the vagina, being slightly ridged or bumpy.

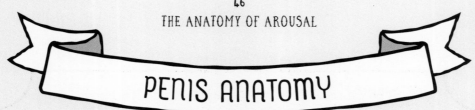

PENIS ANATOMY

It is possible to have lots of pleasure without an erection, and sensual massage, partnered or solo, is a great opportunity to experiment with that. You might get and lose an erection in a massage, or you might never become erect at all. All of it is normal. See what feels genuinely good and interesting to you, learn how to vary your touch and communicate about it; this can open up a whole new world of sensation for you!

External penis anatomy

While it might be a short tour, there's a lot to say when it comes to touching the external genitals of penis owners. Get comfortable and tune into your sensations as you begin to map your genitals.

THE FRENULUM AND CORONAL RIDGE

While the **glans**, or head, of the penis is often the most sensitive area, there can be hidden, surprisingly sensitive areas that go unexplored. Spend time exploring the **frenulum** and the **coronal ridge**. The frenulum is located on the underside of the glans and on an uncircumcised penis it is where the foreskin connects to the shaft. The coronal ridge is the underside of the "mushroom cap" shape of the glans. They're more pronounced when the penis is erect, but can also be explored while it is soft. Use a lubricated fingertip to map both structures and see if you notice any particularly sensitive areas.

THE SCROTUM AND TESTICLES

Extending down from the base of the shaft of the penis, the **scrotum** is a protective sac that encloses the **testicles**. Many penis owners are surprised to find that manipulating this tissue can be very pleasurable; try gently stretching, massaging, and rolling the skin in your hands. The testicles, two organs responsible for sperm production, can also be pleasurable when played with lightly; try cupping them with your palm, rolling, and massaging them.

PERINEUM

As with vulva owners, the **perineum** is an important area for pelvic and sexual health. It can also be very sensational to massage given its proximity to the prostate gland on the inside of the pelvis. Locate between the scrotum and the anus, then apply pressure to the perineum, massaging in circles or pressing gently in toward your pelvis. The bulb, or root, of the penis also attaches here and becomes tangibly erect during arousal and pleasurable to massage.

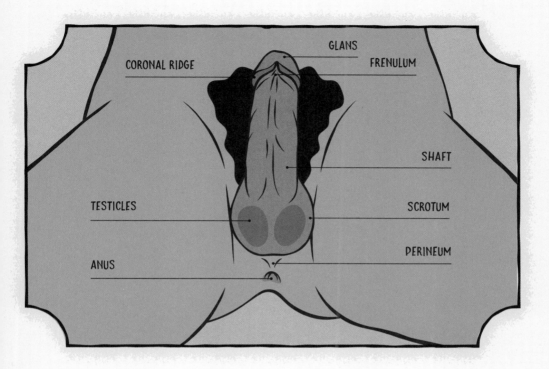

CORONAL RIDGE

GLANS

FRENULUM

SHAFT

TESTICLES

SCROTUM

PERINEUM

ANUS

Internal penis anatomy

Moving on to the internal exploration, if you are following along with your hands, I recommend proceeding with trimmed fingernails, plenty of lubrication, and a spirit of patience and curiosity.

THE PROSTATE GLAND

The walnut-shaped prostate gland is located behind the front wall of the rectum, toward the belly, about a finger's length inside the anal canal. Due to its internal location and the lingering taboo around anal stimulation, many penis owners do not explore the potential pleasure of their prostate gland. While its main function is the production of sperm, it's also an erogenous zone that can be incredibly powerful when included in a massage or sexual exchange. If anal exploration is new to you and you're wondering where to start, don't fret; there's a whole section dedicated to that coming up (see pages 48–49). In general, gentle stroking rather than poking is best here.

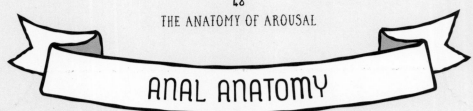

ANAL ANATOMY

In general, anal sphincters are not to be rushed. They are incredibly responsive, but approach them slowly and with sensitivity and your explorations will yield more information and sensation.

To begin familiarizing yourself with your anus, consider exploring its external surface in the shower or bath where you'll feel clean and relaxed. Don't insert soap into the anus, as that can be very irritating. If you have a vagina, please remember never to put any finger or object that's been in contact with your anus into your vagina to avoid infection.

Outside of the shower or bath, it's useful to have some disposable gloves or skin-friendly disinfectant wipes and lubricant on hand. The anal canal and rectum do not self-lubricate, so body-safe oils and lubricants are your friend in this situation. Don't hesitate to use them. Find a position that is comfortable, either on your side or on your back with your knees bent.

External anal exploration

First, just explore the texture and sensation of the external surface of the anus. This is the **external anal sphincter**, which is made up of voluntary muscle and therefore under conscious control. It is one area of the pelvic muscles that most people find easier to contract and relax; try pulling the sphincter up and away from your finger and you'll be contracting the muscles. Gently bear down and push the sphincter toward your finger to expand them.

These muscles can be chronically tense due to many factors. If you notice excess tension here, try breathing slowly and deeply into your abdomen and pelvis. See if the external anal sphincter can soften and expand on your inhale. The more you practice this, the more relaxed your anus and entire pelvis can become. This sphincter is rich in nerve endings, so tune into your sensations as you explore it. What do you notice?

During arousal, in all people, the blood vessels and erectile tissue in this area swell and darken in color. The muscles connected to the external sphincter contribute to the contractions that make arousal and orgasm pleasurable. The many nerve endings here and in the perineal area make external anal touch very sensational during sensual and sexual play.

Internal anal exploration

Just inside the external anal sphincter is the **anal canal** and the **internal anal sphincter**. The anal canal is a tubelike structure whose folded layers of tissue give it a remarkable capacity to expand. It is more sensitive to pressure than touch. About an inch in length, it is capped by the internal anal sphincter. This internal sphincter is controlled by involuntary

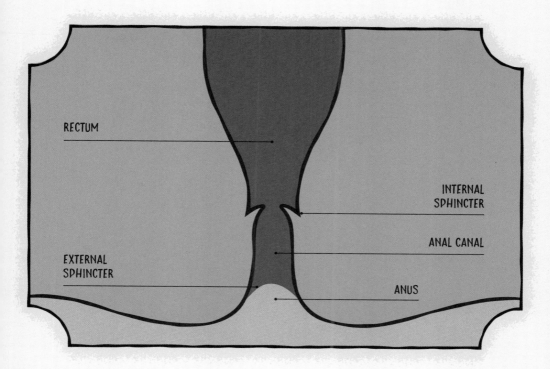

RECTUM

INTERNAL
SPHINCTER

ANAL CANAL

EXTERNAL
SPHINCTER

ANUS

muscles, so it is not under conscious control. Nevertheless, it is possible to help it relax via deep breathing and slow, sensitive touch.

In penis owners, internal anal touch may be pleasurable due to the proximity of the root of the penis to the prostate gland. Pleasurable internal anal sensation in vulva owners may be due to the proximity of the vestibular bulbs to the rectal walls.

To explore internally, start by breathing deeply into the abdomen and relaxing the external sphincter as much as you can. If you are a vulva owner, be sure to cover the entrance to your vagina with a cloth to avoid any lubricant moving from the anus to the vagina. Slowly insert a well-lubricated finger into the anal canal and move inward until you find the internal sphincter. Some people find it most helpful to simply hold their finger there and breathe, allowing the muscles and sphincter to relax and acclimate to the pressure.

Over time, you can experiment with touching each area of the circular anal canal as if moving hour by hour on a clock face; twelve o'clock facing your belly and six o'clock facing your tailbone. Once your internal anal sphincter is relaxed enough, you can explore past it and into the rectum. Don't push, don't force. Take your time and follow your body's sensations. Commit yourself to not tolerating pain and instead create an experience of curious, potentially pleasurable self-exploration.

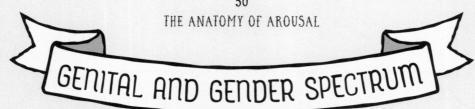

GENITAL AND GENDER SPECTRUM

Gender and genitals are a fascinating and complex subject.
Traditionally, our education begins and ends with a very strict
binary: female and male, vulvas and penises, and that's it. In reality,
there is a spectrum of genders and genital presentations.

Genitals are made up of many interacting physical phenomenon—genetics, sex hormones, and physical presentation. Gender is shaped by the ways we are raised, society's expectations, personal awareness, self-discovery, and choice. When a doctor holds a newborn baby, they only see the external genitals and decide whether it will be F or M that goes on the birth certificate. But as society evolves to include a more broad definition of gender, we see that this approach is limiting.

Intersex is a general description of anyone who is born with genitals that don't fit the standard, medical definition of female or male. This can take on myriad presentations, some quite typical and some quite different. I mention it here in an effort to bring more awareness to the immense, natural variation of human genital anatomy and normalize an otherwise hush-hush topic. If you or anyone you exchange a massage with has genitals presenting outside of the standard F and M categories, it only takes an open discussion about what language preferences you each have for your genitals to proceed as usual.

The same approach goes for non-binary and transgender genital owners. **Non-binary** people identify themselves outside of the gender binary, neither female nor male. They may refer to their genitals outside the vulva and penis binary as well, and have different names and needs regarding their treatment.

Transgender genitals can change dramatically if a person has decided to have hormone therapy or surgery. Even if not, they may want their genitals referred to in alignment with their gender identity, or something else entirely. Again, it comes down to having an open mind, an honest conversation, and a spirit of curiosity.

No matter what kind of body you have, a sensual massage can be a wonderful way to connect more deeply with every part of it and bring acceptance, compassion, and knowledge to your genitals in particular.

HELPFUL QUESTIONS

These questions may help you negotiate and learn
from your explorations of your pleasure anatomy.

WHAT AREAS OF YOUR GENITALS DID YOU
NOTICE FELT PARTICULARLY GOOD?

. . . .

DID ANY AREA OF YOUR GENITALS SURPRISE
YOU WITH UNEXPECTED SENSATION?

. . . .

IS THERE A PART OF YOUR GENITALS
YOU'D LIKE TO EXPLORE MORE?

. . . .

HOW CAN YOU INCORPORATE MORE CURIOSITY
AND EXPERIMENTATION INTO TOUCHING YOUR GENITALS?

THE BODY IS AN INSTRUMENT WHICH
ONLY GIVES OFF MUSIC WHEN IT IS USED
AS A BODY. ALWAYS AN ORCHESTRA, AND
JUST AS MUSIC TRAVERSES WALLS, SO
SENSUALITY TRAVERSES THE BODY AND
REACHES UP TO ECSTASY.

Anais Nin

CHAPTER 4

YOUR SENSUAL MASSAGE TOOLBOX

There are many ways to enhance your sensual massage experience, customizing each aspect to better please yourself and your partner. It doesn't require an expensive shopping trip either, as you may already have plenty of tools in your home that can make your massage even more perfect.

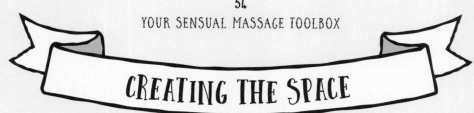

CREATING THE SPACE

The space in which you choose to give and receive your massage is just as important as the massage itself. Our environments have a huge impact on our minds and emotions.

Remember how the brain is scanning your environment for threat (see page 16)? Well, a messy, uninviting room could actually tip it off, along with inadequate privacy, uncomfortable temperatures, etc. Your massage is special, private, and sensual. It is best if your space reflects those same ideas. It doesn't take remodeling, just a commitment to your and your partner's comfort and pleasure.

Physical environment

Find ways to incorporate all of your senses to create a fully immersive experience.

- Put aside enough time to slow down and drop into the experience.
- Make sure your space is secure and you won't be interrupted.
- Do you prefer it warm or cool? Set the temperature to your comfort level.
- Consider dimming the lights with colorful silk cloths or lighting candles with sumptuous scents.
- Choose music that is soothing and won't distract you, or cue up nature sounds, or, if it's available outside, open the window and let nature's music come to you.
- If you are receiving, choose colors and textures to lie on that you most enjoy.

Emotional environment

Creating the space may sometimes require clearing the air. If there are difficulties or resentments from the day lingering between you and your partner, it can make it hard to fully relax. You may not be able to resolve everything before a massage, but if you or your partner need to voice any concerns, try doing that before your session in compassionate, nonjudgmental ways.

Focus your communication on how you feel and your own experience, not on what your partner has or hasn't done, which may take a much longer conversation to address. Being honest about your current feelings without trying to fix the cause of them right this moment can help you to unburden your heart, relax your body, and connect with your partner.

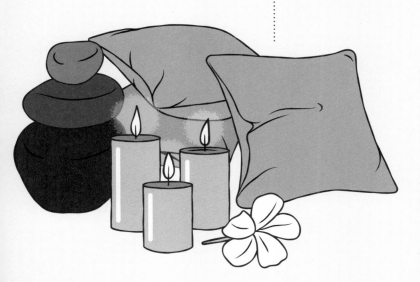

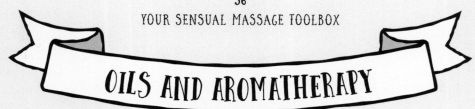

OILS AND AROMATHERAPY

There are innumerable body-safe oils and creams to choose from these days, as a stroll down any aisle in a body care store will show you. In general, you want to use something that won't be absorbed too quickly by the skin, which many creams are designed to do, so I personally prefer to use oil.

Base massage oils

The lighter the oil, the faster it absorbs, but it is also less likely to leave stains or an overly sticky feeling on the skin. The heavier the oil, the less you have to use in order to glide on the skin, but you do run the risk of leaving some stains on your sheets.

LIGHTER OILS

Oils on the lighter side include **grapeseed** oil, a great choice for anyone with sensitive skin, and **almond** oil, which is good so long as you or your partner don't have a nut allergy.

HEAVIER OILS

On the heavier side are **jojoba** oil and **coconut** oil, both of which are wonderful for dry skin.

OILS FOR INTERNAL USE

For internal use, I prefer **coconut** oil or **castor** oil. Castor oil is very viscous so a little goes a long way, and it has remarkable healing properties, including being antibacterial and antifungal. Be warned, however, castor oil can definitely leave stains.

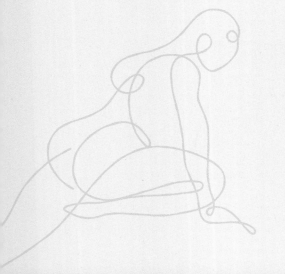

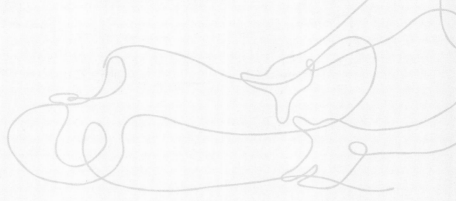

Essential oils

Aromatherapy is based on using essential oils and other aromatic compounds—mixed in with the base oil—during a massage. Smell is our oldest sense and it bypasses our conscious mind to go straight to our evolutionarily "older" brain, the area that is most concerned with safety. Incorporating even a small amount of a soothing scent can greatly enhance your ability to relax.

Included here are some recipes for you to try, but feel free to create your own combinations. Remember never to use essential oils directly on the skin; instead, mix them with a carrier oil—the **essential oil content** should make up **2%** of the mix, so up to 13 drops to 1 oz (30 ml) of base oil.

EXTERNAL USE ONLY
Essential oils are **not appropriate for internal use**, even when combined with a base oil.

Tranquillity blend

8 drops lavender essential oil
5 drops clary sage essential oil
7 drops lemon essential oil

Passion blend

6 drops ginger essential oil
6 drops orange essential oil

Seduction blend

6 drops rose essential oil
4 drops ylang ylang essential oil
6 drops lemon essential oil

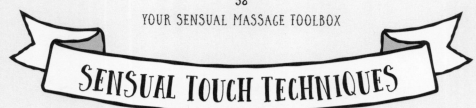

SENSUAL TOUCH TECHNIQUES

Sensual massage is the practice of touching your partner or yourself in a way that elicits pleasure, which is always unique to the moment, and using traditional massage techniques.

These traditional techniques can help lend your massage a sense of flow and are excellent for increasing circulation and relaxation. They are very easy to blend with less traditional, more sensual techniques, as it only takes a simple change in the way you're using your hands.

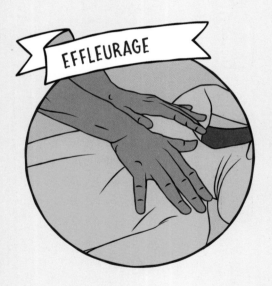

EFFLEURAGE

Traditional

Effleurage strokes are **long** and **gliding**, with open, flat palms that move the oil all over the body part you are massaging. This is a perfect "opening" and "closing" stroke.

Sensual

You can also **stroke** lightly with the **fingertips**. It can be ticklish, but sometimes the softer touches can create the biggest sensations.

- Gliding
- Sliding
- Dragging
- Stroking

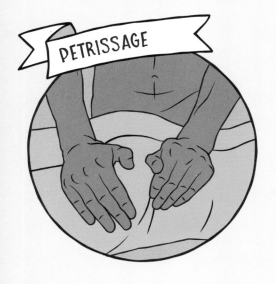

PETRISSAGE

Traditional

Also called **kneading**, this stroke goes below the skin layer and moves the fascia and muscle tissue with your palms and fingers.

Sensual

You can **squeeze** and **grasp** the muscle tissue for a more intense, possessive effect.

- Kneading
- Compressing
- Squeezing
- Pressing
- Pinching

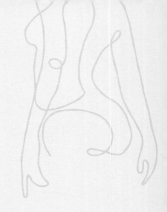

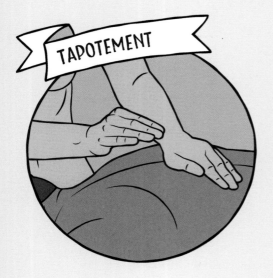

TAPOTEMENT

Traditional

A very **invigorating** technique, this is best used when you want to increase the energy and "wake up" the skin. With loosely cupped palms or closed fists, you rhythmically tap the skin deep enough to contact the fascia and muscle layer but not so deep as to cause pain. This works best on thicker, more fleshy parts of the body, but can be applied lightly to thinner areas as well.

Sensual

Scratching, lightly dragging your fingernails across the skin, or using them to scratch the scalp, can be very sensational.

Spanking is the adult cousin of tapotement. Try this on the thicker parts of the body like the buttocks and thighs. Experiment with quickly removing your hand or leaving it on the skin and notice the difference.

- Tapping
- Shaking
- Scratching
- Spanking

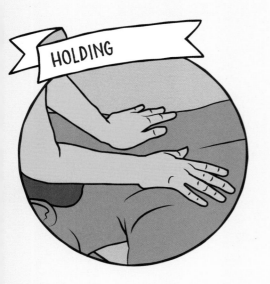

HOLDING

Sometimes, stillness is a technique all its own. Simply holding a part of the body still in your hands with awareness and care can be very nurturing and grounding.

- Holding
- Breathing
- Resting

BODY TOUCH

Don't be afraid to explore using more of your body than just your hands. Your forearms, feet, hair, breath, lips, and tongue are all available in your sensual toolbox as well. Just remember to communicate with your partner about what feels best and what you'd like to try. Stay curious and you can't go wrong!

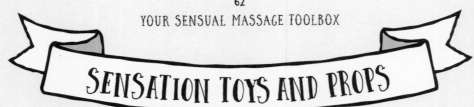

SENSATION TOYS AND PROPS

A massage is a great opportunity to explore using objects and toys to create different sensations. Turn a creative eye on your household and ask yourself what you could incorporate into your massage? Or take a trip to a sex shop for some dedicated tools. Either way, remember to provide contrast with whatever you choose to play with and follow your pleasure.

Textures and temperatures

Think back to the exercises on pages 28–33, and the sensations you've discovered that you enjoy. What do you have at home to help you create them during your massage?

- You might have an ice pack and hot-water bottle for playing with **temperatures**.
- You probably have some very **soft** fabrics or silks, loofahs, or sponges to play with soft and **rough** sensations.
- Bags of beans or rice or a weighted blanket are great options to play with **weight**.

In a shop you'll find myriad vibrators, feathers, pinwheels, paddles, floggers, and massage tools to keep you experimenting for a lifetime.

Comfort

Props are also very useful in a massage. This could mean lots of **pillows**, **bolsters**, and **blankets**, or specially designed wedges and bolsters found in sex shops. If you need extra support for any part of your body, don't hesitate to acquire it. You want to be as comfortable as possible so you can fully relax. No, you're not "needy" or "taking too much" if you require lots of support! You're just committing yourself to a special experience geared toward pleasure and relaxation.

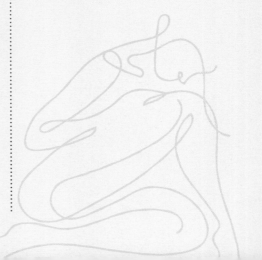

HELPFUL QUESTIONS

These questions may help you to understand what it is you need to feel safe, open, and relaxed before you begin a massage.

THINK OF SENSATIONS YOU MOST ENJOY, ARE THERE TOOLS YOU HAVE AT HOME THAT YOU COULD USE TO RECREATE THEM?

....

HOW CAN YOU CREATE CONTRASTING SENSATIONS DURING YOUR MASSAGE?

....

HOW CAN YOU INVOLVE EACH OF YOUR SENSES DURING YOUR MASSAGE?

....

HOW MANY DIFFERENT PARTS OF YOUR HANDS OR YOUR BODY CAN YOU EXPERIMENT WITH IN THE MASSAGE?

AS TOUCH OPENS THE HEART AND SOOTHES
THE CHATTERING MIND . . . IT SUPPORTS
VALUES THAT EMERGE FROM THE
EXPERIENCE OF PLEASURE: GRATITUDE, JOY,
FORGIVENESS, CONNECTION, COMPASSION.

Caffyn Jesse

CHAPTER 5

ALL TOGETHER NOW

Now that you've spent some time getting to know your boundaries, creating consent, increasing your pleasure awareness, learning about your anatomy, and adding to your sensation toolbox, it's time to put it all together and embark on your sensual massage adventure. Here you will find suggestions for how to open and close your session and a step-by-step guide that you can follow entirely or simply use for guidance and inspiration.

OPENING YOUR PRACTICE

Before jumping into your session, take a moment to sit with your partner. If you are giving the massage, ask the other if there's anything they'd like to talk about or request from you before starting. If you are receiving the massage, take this time to establish any boundaries and make any requests or adjustments to your space that you need to feel most comfortable and safe.

Together, set an intention for your session. It could be to feel more connected to one another, to experience your own and each other's bodies in a new way, or simply to have fun! You can also set individual intentions and share them with one another. Perhaps as the giver your intention could be to stay attuned to your partner and create a safe space for them. As the receiver your intention might be to follow your pleasure and ask for exactly what you want.

Finally, spend just a few minutes breathing together. If possible, sync your breathing with your partner's. This has a connecting and grounding effect, a perfect state in which to start your massage.

See also

BOUNDARIES AND CONSENT: PAGES 16–25

THE PATH TO PLEASURE: PAGES 28–37

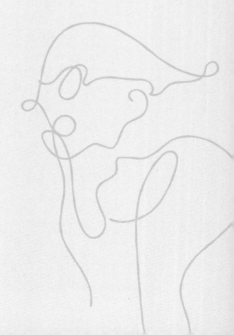

OPENING YOUR PRACTICE

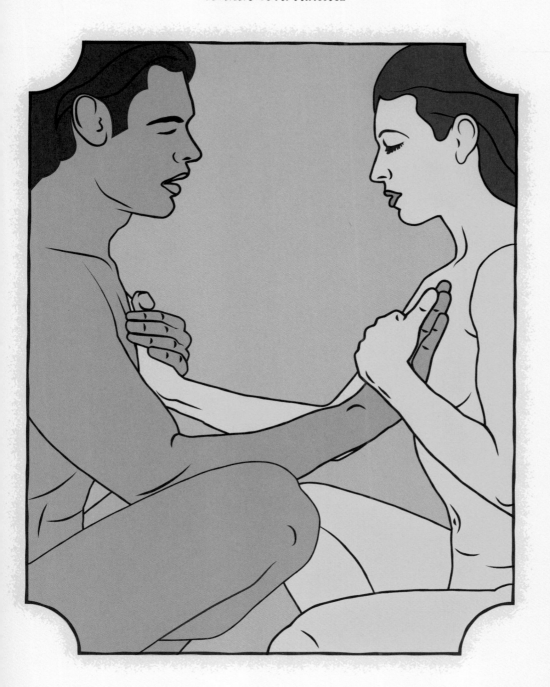

BACK AND HIPS

The back is a wonderful place to start your sensual massage. Be it in the neck or upper or lower back, this area of complex muscle intersections can be a repository of both mental and physical stress. Including the muscles of the hips is important since tension around these joints often directly contributes to our experience of back pain, and can lead to less blood circulation in the pelvis—a very important area of arousal!

Beginning with a "tertiary" erogenous zone (while there is no hierarchy, it is useful to organize these zones into primary, secondary, and tertiary) is a good way to warm up toward working on your partner's more sensitive erogenous zones. It also helps to create relaxation, which increases arousal and fosters a supportive, connected experience. Men, women, and non-binary folks can all experience a great deal of sensual pleasure from a massage in this area. Just remember to explore with curiosity, ask open-ended questions, and have fun.

Sensual touch techniques

EFFLEURAGE: PAGE 58
Stroking; dragging; gliding; sliding

PETRISSAGE: PAGE 59
Squeezing; kneading; pressing

TAPOTEMENT: PAGE 60
Scratching; shaking; spanking

HOLDING: PAGE 61
Breathing

See also

CREATING THE SPACE: PAGES 54-55

OILS AND AROMATHERAPY: PAGES 56-57

SENSATION TOYS AND PROPS: PAGE 62

SACRUM

GLUTEAL CLEFT

HIP

THIGH

SEQUENCE FOR BACK

①

Start at your partner's head. Rest your hands on their shoulders and take a moment to tune into their breath. It might be obvious or subtle; just try to sense any movement underneath your hands. As they exhale, stroke your palms down either side of their spine to just above where their hips begin.

②

Drag or **scratch** your fingers back up, either lightly over the spine or deeper on either side. Include the back of their neck and head; run your fingers through their hair, **stroke** the sensitive area just below the ear, **squeeze** the muscles of their neck, or try using your breath here, too.

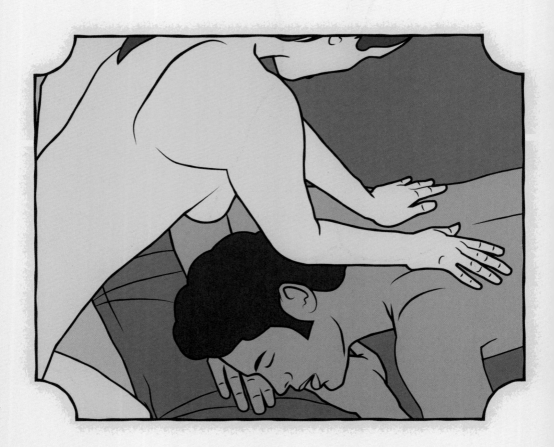

Incorporate other parts of your body to touch
up and down the back—you can use your hair,
different parts of your hands, your forearms,
your lips, your tongue, for example.

Repeat Steps 1–3 as many times as
your partner desires, experimenting with
different touch techniques or incorporating
sensation tools.

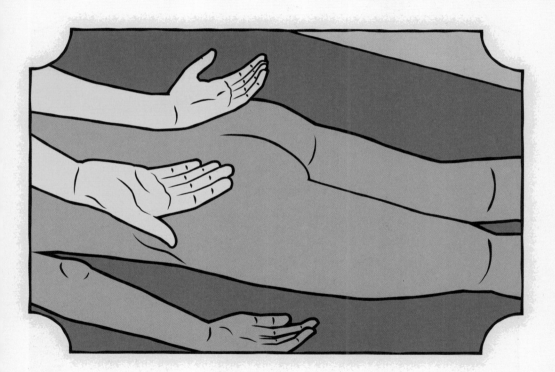

SENSATION TOOLS

Choose a few sensation tools and experiment with contrast—start with something smooth,
then try something rough, and go from cool to warm temperatures, etc. Gradually increase
the intensity of the sensations. Watch and listen to your partner for cues of their relaxation
and enjoyment. Remember: when in doubt, ask for feedback!

Sitting beside your partner, place your hands on their body. **Knead** the muscles just beside their spine with the heel of your hands, working up and down the length of their back.

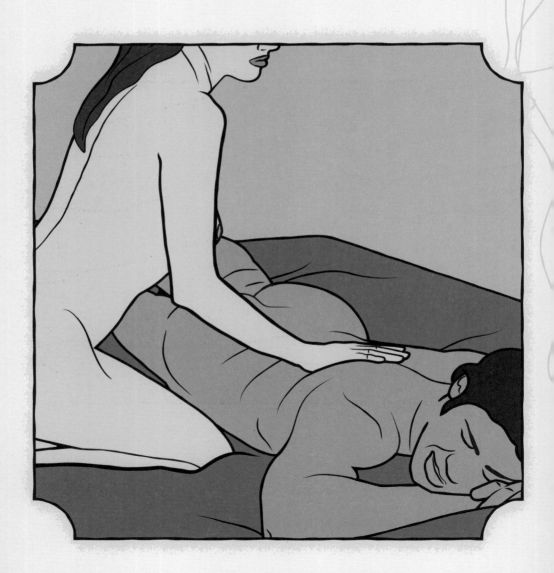

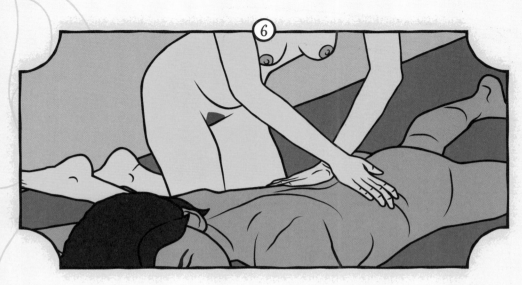

Starting at the lower back, place one hand on your partner's opposite side and your other hand on the side closest to you. Draw your hands toward one another, dragging the muscles underneath toward the center. **Glide** gently over the spine as your hands pass one another and move a few inches up your partner's body; continue to travel upward in this "X" pattern.

With both hands on the opposite side, try pulling their body toward you and gently dropping it back down to create a rocking motion in their torso. This gentle, wavelike motion can do wonders to relax the whole nervous system of your partner.

Stroke, **squeeze**, **drag**, and **scratch** their flank. Include the sides of the belly, chest, and armpit. These areas can be ticklish but also exquisitely sensitive.

Repeat Steps 5–8 on each side as much as your partner desires, experimenting with different kinds of touch and using your sensation tools.

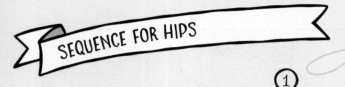

SEQUENCE FOR HIPS

①

Position yourself between your partner's legs, facing their back. **Knead** both buttocks with your hands in soft fists. Pay attention to areas of tension on either side of the sacrum (the triangular bone found at the base of the spine), and try **kneading**, **squeezing**, and **dragging** your fingertips over these tense spots.

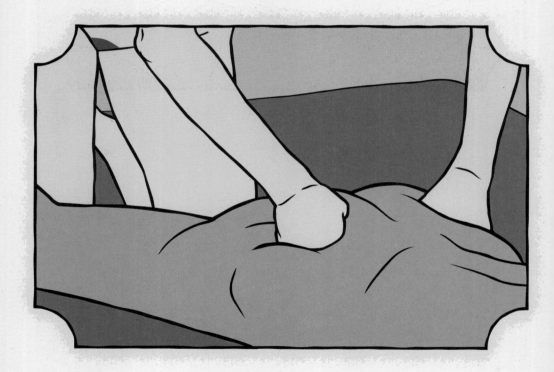

Experiment with **shaking**, squeezing different parts of the hips, and moving the tissue in different directions. This helps loosen the muscles and increase circulation to the pelvis, a crucial element in physiological arousal.

BACK AND HIPS

③

Play with impact and pressure; try **spanking** the glutes and the backs of the thighs. Experiment with following the spanking with a **hold**, or immediately remove your hand and see which your partner likes best. Avoid impact directly on the sacrum bone. Since there are a lot of important nerves that travel through this bone, it can be a surprisingly sensitive area. Try lightly **kneading**, or **stroking** fingertips instead.

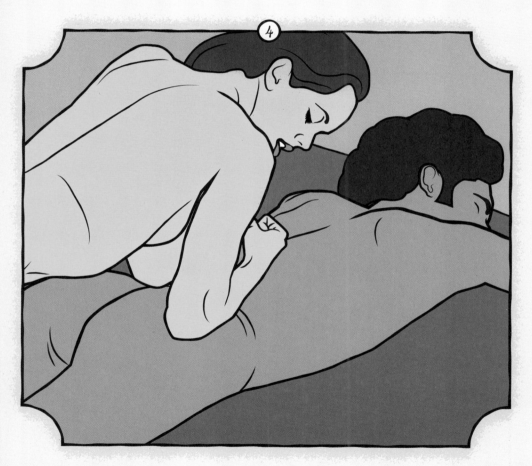

As with the back sequence, see how many parts of your body you can incorporate into the massage of this area. If you've already played with impact, try playing with a gentle sensation tool such as a silk scarf, a soft mitt, your hair, or your relaxed tongue.

Include the area in between the gluteal cleft. Trying stroking, dragging, and light kneading here. Include the perineum, which can help relax the whole pelvic floor.

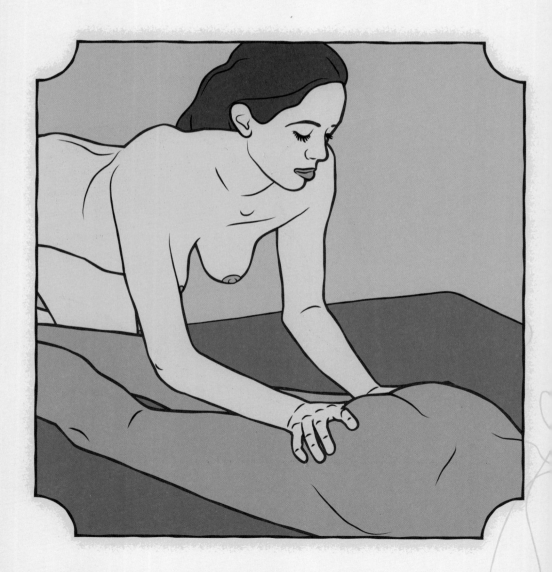

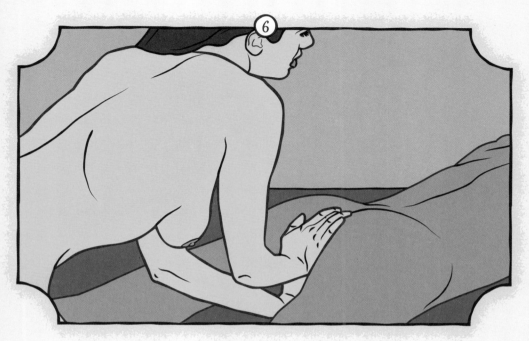

If including anal touch, you can drag the pinky edge of your palms over the external anal sphincter, either one at a time or simultaneously, and use your fingertips to stroke the external anal sphincter.

⑦

Use your fingertips to gently circle, **press** into, and stretch the external sphincter of the anus. A vibrator can be wonderful here, but remember that sphincters are very sensitive and don't like to be rushed! Consistent, gradually increased pressure is best.

ESSENTIAL HYGIENE FOR ANAL TOUCH

As the giving partner, use gloves if you have any cuts or scrapes on your fingers or cuticles. Be careful to separate touching your partner's anus and touching the rest of their body, so you don't spread any bacteria that may be in the area of their anus.

If the receiving partner has internal genitalia, place a barrier, such as a clean cloth, between it and their anus in case any oil or bacteria migrate during the massage.

BACK OF LEGS AND FEET

Moving down from the back and the hips, we end the massage of the
back body on the legs and feet. While not generally considered erotic,
these parts of our bodies can often hide some delightful erogenous
zones; the backs of the knees and soles of the feet, to name just a few.
The rest you will discover for yourself!

This is an area of the body where muscle
tension contributes to back and hip pain, since
shortness in the calves and hamstrings can pull
on the muscles above and create more stress.
Massaging the muscle groups in the thighs, lower
legs, and feet can help the rest of the body relax.
The broader surface of the thighs also provides
a great space to play with your impact and
sensation tools.

Sensual touch techniques

EFFLEURAGE: PAGE 58
Stroking

PETRISSAGE: PAGE 59
Compressing; kneading; squeezing; pressing

TAPOTEMENT: PAGE 60
Scratching; spanking

HOLDING: PAGE 61
Resting

See also

CREATING THE SPACE: PAGES 54-55

OILS AND AROMATHERAPY: PAGES 56-57

SENSATION TOYS AND PROPS: PAGE 62

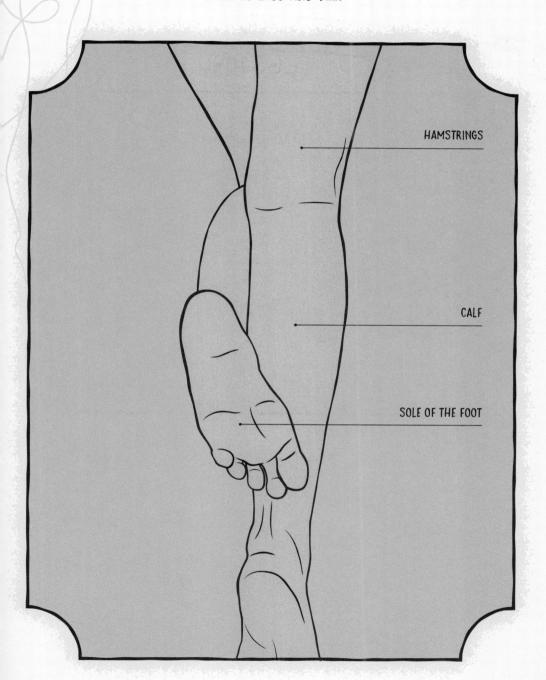

HAMSTRINGS

CALF

SOLE OF THE FOOT

SEQUENCE FOR BACK OF THE LEGS

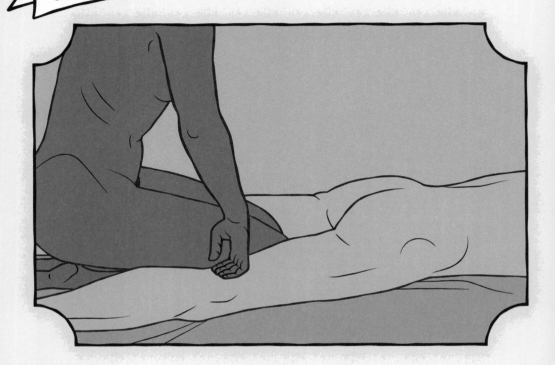

Sit between your partner's knees and place your hands on the upper portion of their thighs. Imagine three lines of muscles running parallel to each other down to their knee; this is the direction and placement of the hamstring muscles. Begin to **compress** these lines up and down between the hip and the knee with your palms. Stretch the tissue away from the midline of the body.

Now that you've warmed up the area, play with **stroking** your fingertips or **scratching** your fingernails up and down the direction of the muscles. Include light touch along the inner thigh; this area can be highly sensitive.

Move your body down to sit between your partner's feet and place your hands on the upper portion of their calves. This time, imagine two lines that run parallel down to the ankle; that is the direction and placement of the calf muscles. **Knead** the calf muscles up and down between the ankle and the knee.

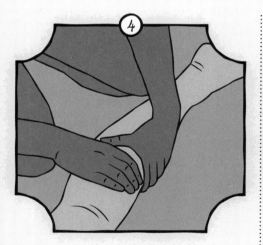

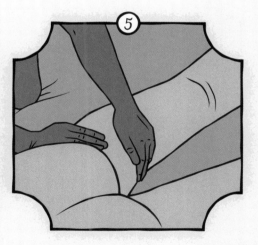

Position yourself so you are sitting outside of one of your partner's legs, in front of their calf muscle. Place your hands around the calf muscle on opposite sides. Pull one hand toward you and push the other away, allowing the hands to pass each other, **squeezing** the muscles in between them. Squeeze down to the ankle and back up again.

Tie in the whole area by squeezing the entire leg, from ankle to hip and back down again. Repeat Steps 4–5 on the other leg.

SEQUENCE FOR SOLES OF THE FEET

Position yourself so your partner's feet are in front of you. Make a loose fist with one hand and press into the sole of the foot with your knuckles. Try this in between the arch and the ball of the foot.

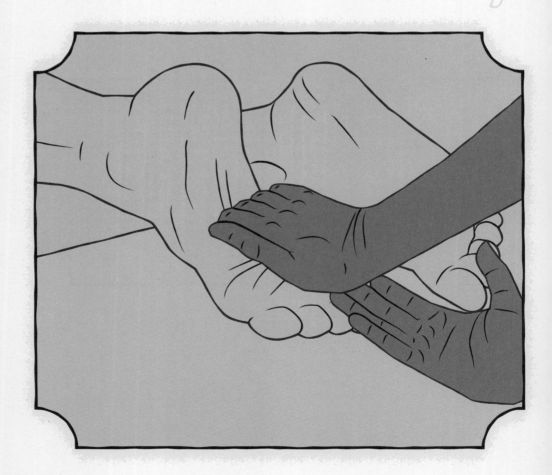

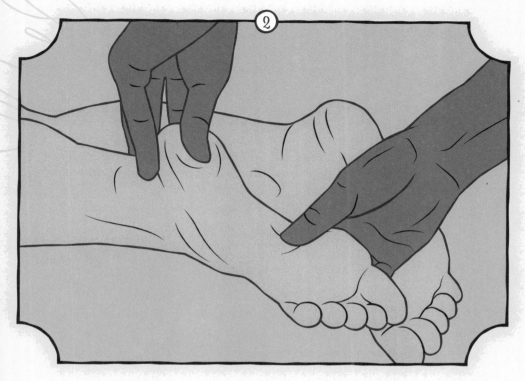

Place the pads of your thumbs on the sole and heel of the foot and wrap your other fingers around the front foot and ankle. Use this hold to gently **knead** circles into the fleshy sole up and down between the heel and the ball of the foot. Repeat Steps 1–2 on the other foot

Now the area should be nice and warm, so try some contrasting sensations, temperatures, and textures. The sole of the foot is incredibly tough and thick, so don't shy away from trying impact or scratching—just be careful of your partner's toes!

Stroke your fingertips down from the heel to the crease of the toes and stroke each individual toe. **Hold** their feet by **resting** the center of your palms on the backs of their heels. Tune into their breath and ground into the present moment before transitioning to the next area of their body.

FACE, NECK, CHEST, AND ARMS

The face, neck, chest, and arms are where we begin the massage for the front of the body. These areas, where the skin is thinner and the muscle groups smaller than on most of the back body, are great for experimenting with lighter and softer touches and tools. So, grab those feathers and silks, fuzzy mittens, and well-worn, favorite sweaters; anything smooth and soft will do.

Your own hands can do wonders here, too, in these tender spaces that are so fragile and hold our intimate organs of expression: our eyes, lips, throats, nipples, hands, etc. Massaging the chest is an opportunity to tune into and match your partner's breathing, a beautiful way to relax and connect to one another. If your partner has had a reconstruction surgery, top surgery, mastectomy, or other surgery in this area it is also a great way to slowly reestablish sensation and circulation, and to address scar tissue. Sometimes our scars can hold a lot of emotional charge, so work sensitively and slowly if this is the case for your partner.

This is very rich territory; I'm excited for you to embark on your explorations!

Sensual touch techniques

EFFLEURAGE: PAGE 58
Stroking; dragging; gliding

PETRISSAGE: PAGE 59
Squeezing; pressing; kneading

TAPOTEMENT: PAGE 60
Shaking

HOLDING: PAGE 61
Breathing

See also

CREATING THE SPACE: PAGES 54-55

OILS AND AROMATHERAPY: PAGES 56-57

SENSATION TOYS AND PROPS: PAGE 62

FACE, NECK, CHEST, AND ARMS

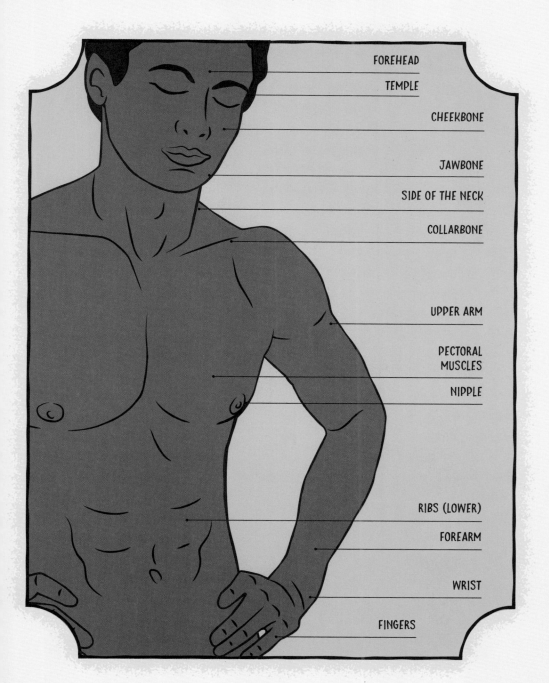

FOREHEAD

TEMPLE

CHEEKBONE

JAWBONE

SIDE OF THE NECK

COLLARBONE

UPPER ARM

PECTORAL MUSCLES

NIPPLE

RIBS (LOWER)

FOREARM

WRIST

FINGERS

SEQUENCE FOR FACE AND NECK

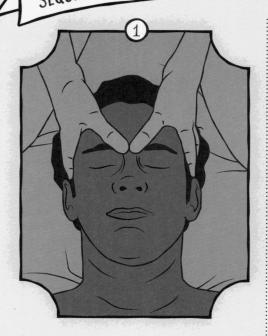

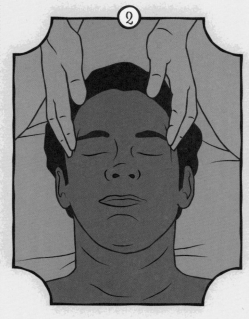

1 With your partner face up, kneel astride their head. Using the pads of your thumbs, stroke a line just between the eyebrows up to the hairline, then follow the hairline down to the temples. On the next pass, stop in the middle of the forehead and **glide** down to the temples. Finally, stroke over the brow bones and eyebrows to the temples.

2 Using the pads of your first and middle fingers, stroke circles over the temples very lightly; this is not the place for deep pressure (although the muscles surrounding it, closer to the ear, can be).

Gently **drag** your fingers over your partner's ears; trace the contours of the shell, **squeeze** the soft cartilage at the bottom, or stretch the tougher cartilage at the top away from the skull. This can be an excellent place to try using your lips, tongue, or **breath**, too!

NATURAL OIL

The skin of the face typically produces enough natural oil to comfortably enhance your touch, so you can set aside your oil until Step 7. If your partner's skin tends toward dryness, use a little moisturizer.

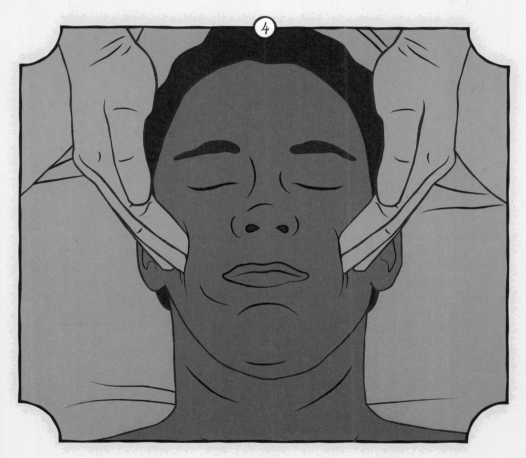

Hook your first three fingers underneath your partner's cheekbones. Drag your fingers along the curve of the bone up toward the temples, then down in the direction of their jawbone. The muscle between the cheekbone and the jawbone, the masseter, is one of the strongest in the body and can hold a lot of tension. Try **pressing** circles into this muscle, up and down the space between the bones.

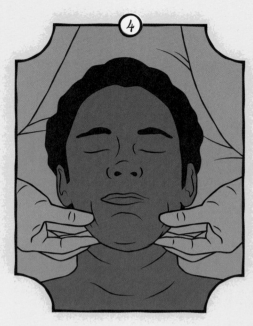

Place your thumb and first finger on the top and the underside of your partner's chin. Squeeze the skin between your fingers, moving out along the jawbone and back in toward the chin.

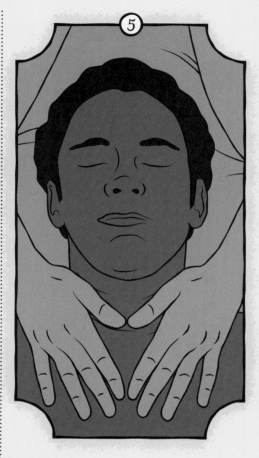

Settle your fingertips on your partner's collarbones; stroke upward along the sides of their neck, over their jawbones, and up to their hairline in one long, smooth motion. Include their hair, brushing it with your fingers or giving it a few gentle tugs to stimulate their scalp.

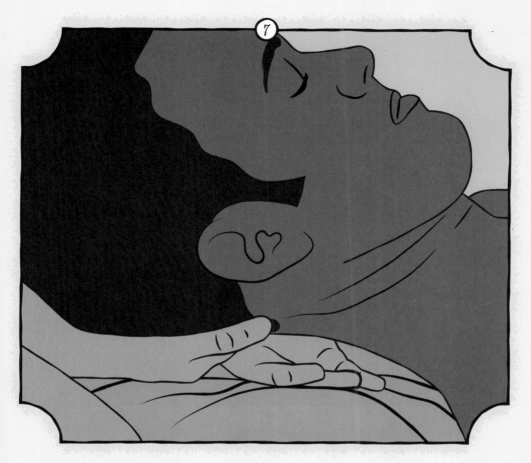

Take your oil and apply some to your hands. With one hand cradling the back of their head, use your other hand to squeeze the muscles of their neck from the top of their shoulders up to the base of their skull. Switch your hands and repeat the same stroke, alternating your hands to create a smooth movement.

Slowly turn their head to one side with your hands. Use the heel of your hand to glide down the side of their neck. Glide your fingertips back up to their skull. Repeat this on the other side.

SEQUENCE FOR CHEST

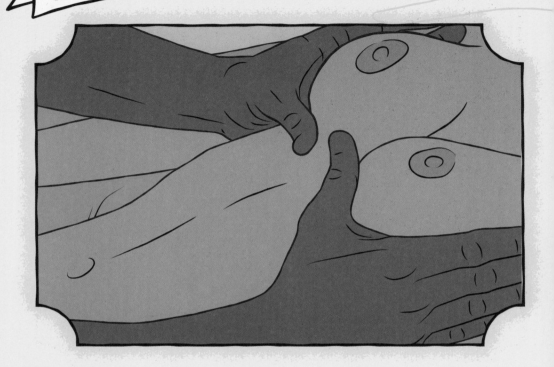

Either straddle your partner's hips or sit to one side of their waist. Place your hands on their lower ribs, taking a moment to feel the movement of their breathing diaphragm underneath your fingers. Glide your palms up between their nipples, over their sternum. Separate your hands at the level of their collarbones and glide them underneath the bone and outward to their pectoral muscles.

Glide your fingertips down to their ribs, outside of their nipples, back to where you started. Imagine you are drawing a heart shape on their chest. Repeat this stroke, starting on their inhale and completing it on their exhale.

Knead one side of their pectoral muscles with the heel of your hand, starting from their sternum and working out to their shoulder and back in again. Repeat on the other side.

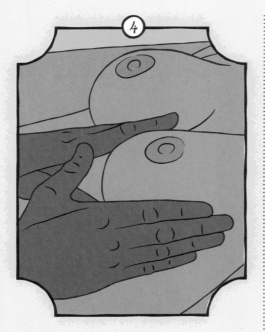

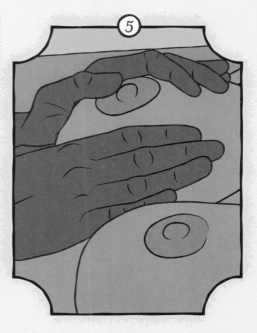

Use both hands on one side of their chest; use your fingertips to knead circles around their breast tissue, spiraling in toward the nipple and spiraling back out again. Avoid direct stimulation of the nipple for now. Trust me, the wait is worth it! Repeat on the other side.

Once the chest area is nice and warmed up, slowly approach the nipple. Less is often more in this area, so I suggest moving slowly and with a soft touch. (Of course, if your partner wants something different, then go with that!) Use the pad of your thumb to lightly flick and circle over the nipple. Your breath, lips, and tongue could be quite sensational here as well. Repeat on the other side.

SEQUENCE FOR ARMS AND HANDS

① Seated to one side of your partner's body, kneel in front of their arm. Hold their hand as if you were giving them a handshake, and lift their forearm up, leaving the elbow on the surface beneath.

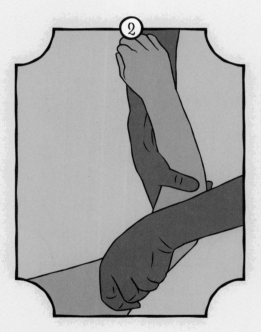

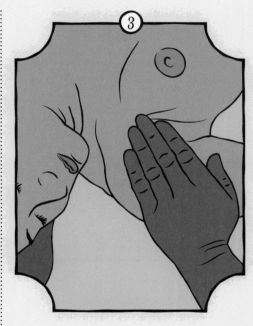

With your four fingers on the underside of their forearm and your thumb on top, squeeze down their arm between their wrist and elbow and back up again.

Drag your palm up your partner's upper arm to their shoulder, kneading circles over the head of their shoulder joint. Glide your fingertips back down to their elbow.

Hold their hand in both of yours with your first four fingers under their palm and your thumbs on top of their hand. Press and drag your fingertips into their palm, then use your thumbs to draw circles over the top of their hand.

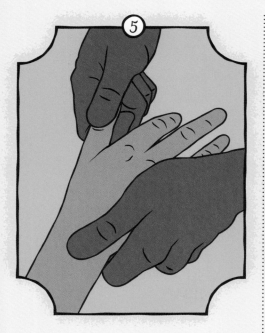

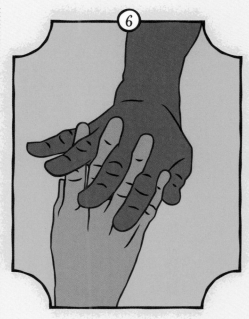

Squeeze each knuckle of your partner's fingers, starting from the base of the pinky finger and working outward.

Intertwine your fingers with theirs and play with shaking their wrist. Using your other hand to hold below their wrist, use your intertwined fingers to move your partner's hand back and forth and in a circle, stretching the wrist joint.

Place their hand back on the surface and use both of your palms to stroke up the entire arm to the shoulder and back down again. Repeat all steps on the other arm.

BELLY AND GENITALS

Moving down from the upper body, we come to massage the abdomen and genitals. This is the literal and figurative core of our body; in Traditional Chinese Medicine this is the energetic center of the body, and in Tantric and Taoist tradition this is where sexual energy arises from, specifically the center of the pelvic floor. This is also the soft, tender home of our visceral, reproductive, and sexual organs.

Unfortunately, many of us absorb negative messages about our bellies from unattainable and unnatural beauty standards, while our genitals are often relegated to complete oblivion, pornographic stereotypes, or the butt of jokes. Ask yourself: how many genitals have you seen besides your own? How often have you taken the time to look at yours? If you're like most people, the answers are not many and not often! That is understandable, and sensual massage is a great (and potentially quite pleasurable!) opportunity to shift the dominant cultural narrative around these misunderstood and maligned parts of ourselves.

As with massaging the rest of the body, but especially for the genitals, touch with curiosity and open-mindedness. Your touch can convey the message that there is no need to perform or react the "right way." The only task is to stay present, notice the sensations, and communicate your needs and desires as they arise, for both the giver and receiver. This is an area that deserves great care and respect, and touching with those values in mind can have a profound impact on a person's sense of connection to themselves and their body.

Sensual touch techniques

EFFLEURAGE: PAGE 58
Gliding; sliding; dragging

PETRISSAGE: PAGE 59
Pressing; kneading; squeezing; pinching

HOLDING: PAGE 61
Resting

See also

CREATING THE SPACE: PAGES 54–55

OILS AND AROMATHERAPY: PAGES 56–57

SENSATION TOYS AND PROPS: PAGE 62

VULVA PLEASURE: PAGES 42–45

PENIS PLEASURE: PAGES 46–47

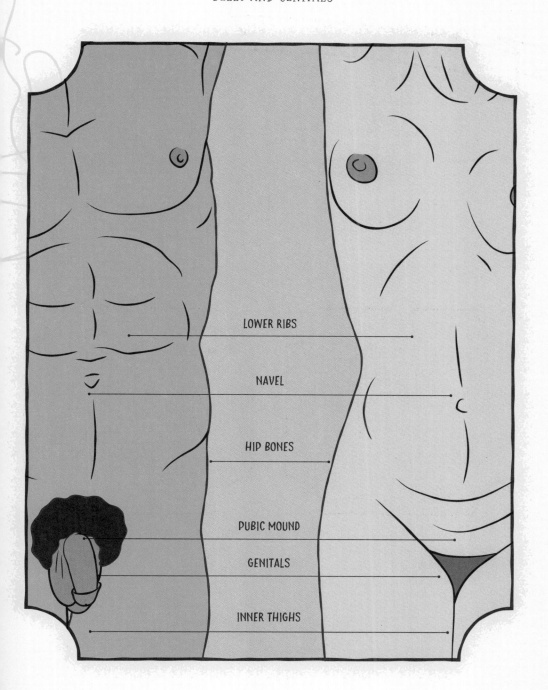

LOWER RIBS

NAVEL

HIP BONES

PUBIC MOUND

GENITALS

INNER THIGHS

SEQUENCE FOR BELLY

①

Kneeling to one side of your partner's hips or between their thighs, rest your palms above their pubic mound, fingers pointing toward their belly button. Ask them to breathe into the space just under your hands and to fully relax their belly. Notice how it expands and contracts underneath your hands. Belly breathing, as it is sometimes called, can be deeply relaxing, and helps to connect the mind to the lower pelvis.

②

Glide your hands up over their belly to the point where their ribs join together. **Press** your fingers into the soft flesh beneath their ribs and **slide** them out to the sides, following just beneath the curve of the ribs.

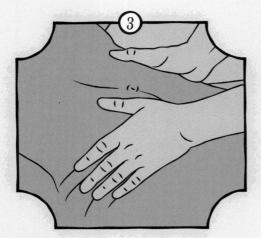

Drag your hands down the sides of the belly to the hips, then together again under the belly button.

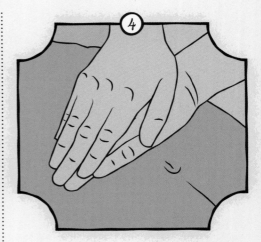

Stack your hands one on top of the other and press small circles all around the navel in a clockwise direction. Spiral your circles outward toward the ribs, hip bones, and pubic mound, then spiral back in toward the navel. Take care not to press too deeply directly over the navel.

Play with **kneading** the soft flesh around the hip area; **squeeze** the sides of the glutes on the outside of the hip bones, or on the space just above them. Knead up to the ribs and back down again on both sides of the belly.

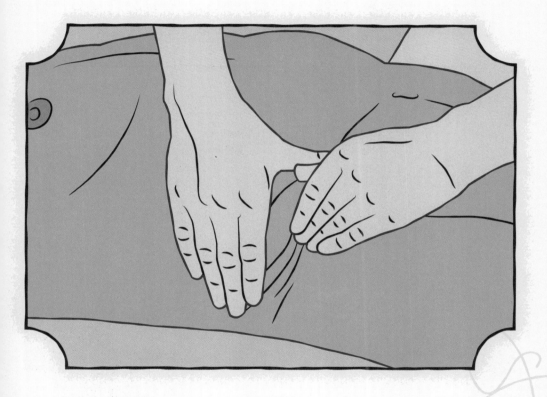

⑥

Finish your belly massage with both hands gliding over the belly in a clockwise direction. Rest your hands above the pubic mound, where you began.

SEQUENCES FOR GENITAL MASSAGE

Here I will outline a few basic sensual strokes for your partner's genitals using the genital configurations of a penis and a vulva. As we discussed in the anatomy chapter, this binary doesn't represent all of the genital spectrum; not even close! That being said, my aim is to make these sequences as adaptable as possible to any set of genitals.

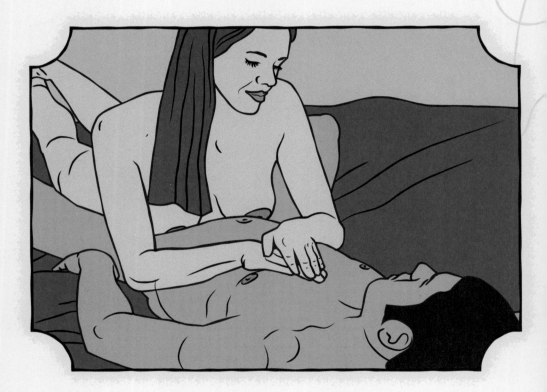

Remember to confirm the language your partner wants to use to address their genitals so you can communicate respectfully. Stay curious and caring and I am sure that whoever you are with and however they present, you can have a marvelous time.

INTERNAL GENITAL ANATOMY

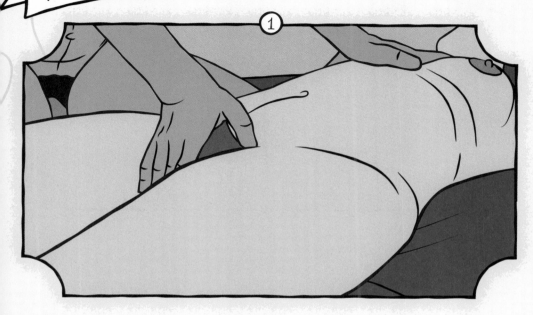

Sit to one side of your partner facing their pelvis. Cup one hand over your partner's groin so your palms and fingers cover their pubic mound and genitals, and rest your other hand on their heart. Holding your partner here is like giving them a hug, sending them warmth and care through your touch. As with the belly massage, encourage your partner to breathe into the space below your hands and notice any movement.

Using your thumb and forefinger, gently **pinch** and **knead** the outer lips on either side of the clitoral hood until they roll out from between your fingers. Work your way down to the perineum and back up again.

Slide your fingers up and down in the deep groove between the inner and outer lips. Circle over the clitoral hood for indirect clitoral stimulation.

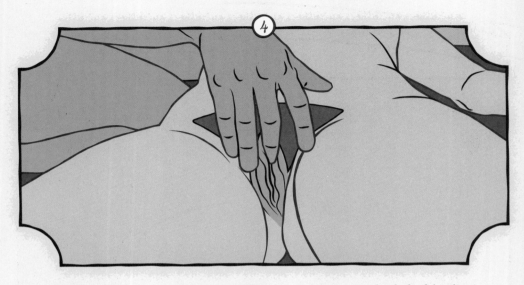

Use your index finger to **drag** the clitoral hood up and down over the shaft of the clitoris.
Press gently on either side of the shaft and see where your partner is more sensitive.

For more direct clitoral stimulation, use plenty of lubrication! With one index finger, pull the clitoral hood up to reveal the head of the clitoris. Experiment with circling over it, **stroking** it from side to side and up and down.

After spending at least ten minutes giving attention to the external genitals, ask for permission to enter their body. You can make the request formal, playful, or even dirty; have fun with it! It's most important that your partner gets a chance to tune in and give you their authentic "yes" or "no."

CLITORAL VIBRATION

If your partner would like to use a vibrator, try cupping your palm over their clitoris and placing the vibrator on your hand. The diffuse vibrations can be wonderful. Much like you approached the head of the clitoris slowly with your fingers, work your way up to direct stimulation with the vibrator. Check in with your partner about the speed and intensity of the vibrator.

If the answer is "yes," stroke the entrance to their vagina or internal genitals. Take your time in this sensitive area to increase sensation and anticipation. Slowly, with plenty of lube, slide one or two fingers inside. Notice the texture, temperature, and subtle movement on the inside of your partner's body. Experiment with slowly moving your fingers in and out, or pressing into the internal walls in four directions, like a gentle stretch. Check in with your partner about what they like best.

To explore the G-crest, curl your fingers toward the top surface of their body and feel for an area that is more wrinkled and spongy than the rest of the canal. Explore which strokes feel best to your partner; maybe it's stroking back and forth, drawing circles, or pressing upward into the tissue. If not fully aroused, this area can be relatively lacking in sensation or even painful. If that is the case now, simply explore a different area and return later, or during another massage session.

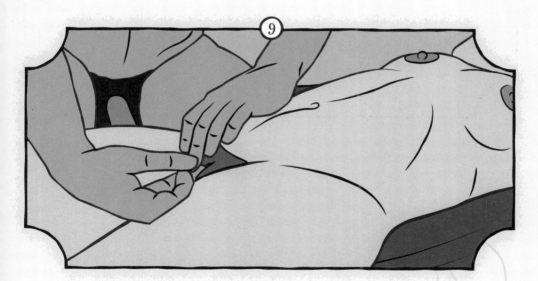

Use your free hand to stimulate your partner's clitoris and play with alternating between clitoral and internal stimulation. Stay in tune with your partner's reactions, energy, and breathing. When in doubt, ask for feedback.

To close, slowly withdraw your fingers and return to the hold from the start of the sequence.

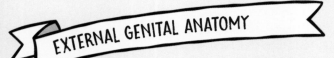

EXTERNAL GENITAL ANATOMY

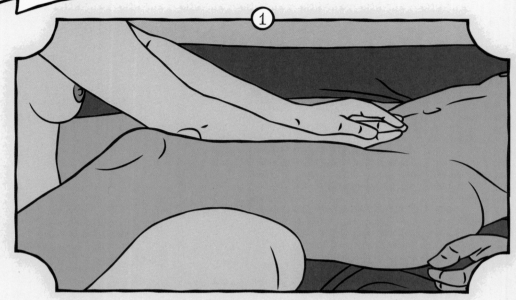

Sit between your partner's legs, draping their thighs over yours. Cup your two hands over their genitals and encourage them to breathe into their lower pelvis and the space underneath your hands.

Hold and **stroke** the shaft of their penis with one hand and knead their perineum with your other hand in a loose fist.

Open your fist and encircle their scrotum with your thumb and index finger. Gently stretch the scrotum away from the body. You can play with stroking the shaft of the penis in the opposite direction, creating a two-way stretch.

Letting go of the scrotum, keep stroking the balls as you stretch the shaft of the penis in a clockwise direction, as if it were the hand of a clock. Take a moment to stroke the shaft at each hour, particularly at six o'clock and twelve o'clock. At the twelve o'clock position, **slide** the flat of your palm up the shaft, over the head, and up your partner's abdomen to their chest. Switch your hands smoothly to create a seamless connection between their genitals and their heart center.

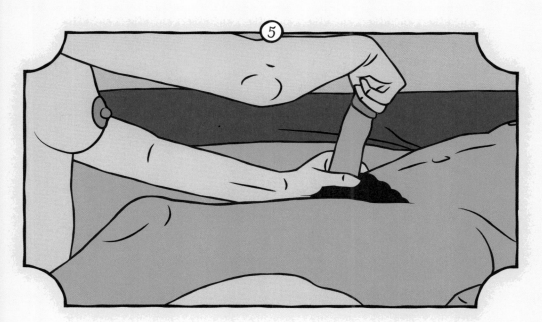

Alternate between stroking the shaft and focusing on the head of the penis. The head of the penis is often the most sensitive area. Alternating between here, the shaft, and the scrotum can help build arousal without tipping over into climax too soon. Twist the shaft and head of the penis as you slide your hand up and down, in a corkscrew motion.

Incorporate your partner's inner thighs, belly, and chest to help spread out the building sexual arousal, and provide varying sensations.

To close, hold one hand still over their genitals and the other over their heart. Take a few breaths together before moving on.

FRONT OF LEGS AND FEET

We'll wrap up our sensual massage journey with the front of the legs and feet. Think of this as a way to ground your partner and bring them back down to earth.

After the potentially ecstatic heights of genital massage, it is important to integrate the rest of the body, reminding your partner that they are a complete, holistic being, with no one part of the body being more or less important than the other.

Like the hamstrings in the back of the thigh, the quadricep muscles in the front can contribute to tension that puts stress on the pelvis and the back. The inner thighs can also benefit from the loosening effects of massage and many people find them quite sensitive. Holding and touching the feet to end the work is a great way to anchor your partner in the present moment, readying them for processing their experience.

Sensual touch techniques

EFFLEURAGE: PAGE 58
Stroking; dragging

PETRISSAGE: PAGE 59
Squeezing; pressing; kneading

HOLDING: PAGE 61
Resting

See also

CREATING THE SPACE: PAGES 54-55

OILS AND AROMATHERAPY: PAGES 56-57

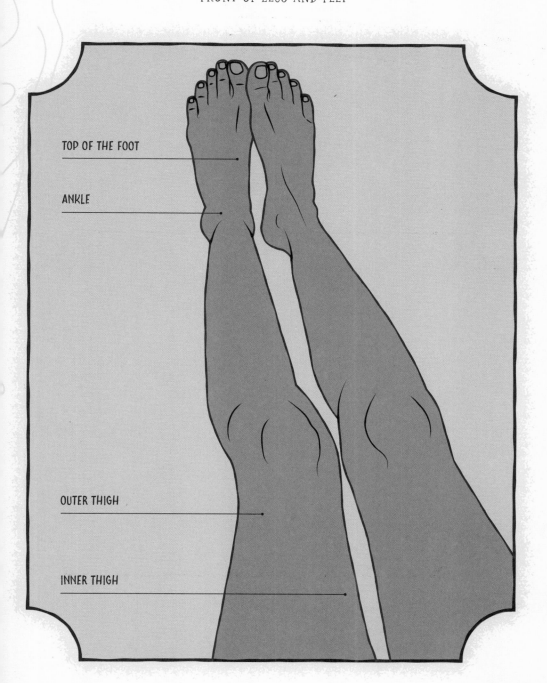

TOP OF THE FOOT

ANKLE

OUTER THIGH

INNER THIGH

SEQUENCE FOR FRONT OF THE LEGS

①

Seated between your partner's legs, place your hands on their upper thighs. **Squeeze** the flesh on the top of their thighs up and down between their hips and knees. Work your way up and down the outer thighs, top of the thighs, and inner thighs.

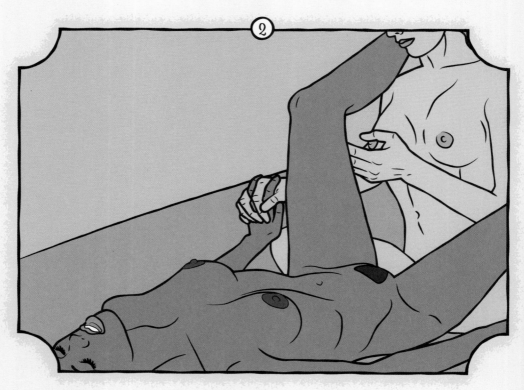

② Place one of their knees on your shoulder to prop their leg up; use this angle to squeeze both the inner and outer thigh, or **stroke** the back of the thigh with your fingertips or fingernails. Repeat with the other leg.

SEQUENCE FOR FRONT OF THE FEET

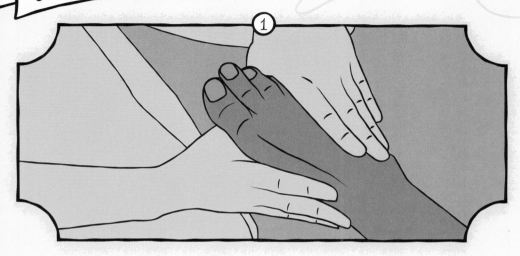

Move down to sit in front of your partner's feet. Use both hands to hold one foot, thumbs on the ball of the foot and the fingertips of the other four fingers on the top surface of the foot. Use the fingers on top to press circles up and down between the toes and the ankle.

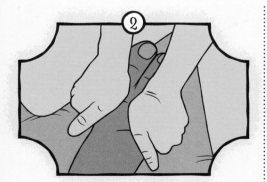

Switch the position of your fingers: thumbs on the top surface, the other four fingers on the bottom surface. **Knead** the top of the foot with the heels of your hands while kneading the bottom of the foot with your fingers.

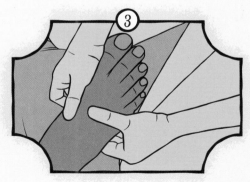

Drag the pads of your thumbs up and down the top surface of the foot and knead circles into the space between the bones of the foot.

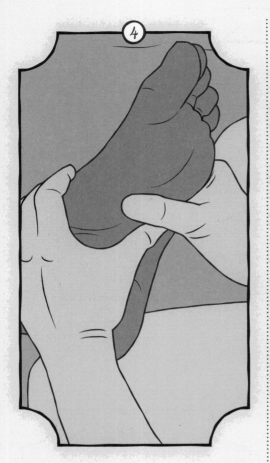

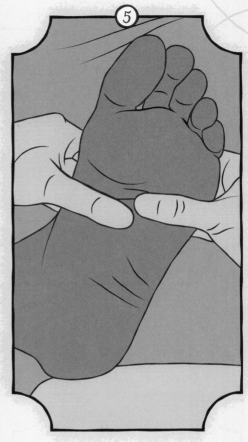

Prop your partner's foot up on your nearest knee; use the pads of your thumbs to press, knead, and drag over the bottom surface of the foot.

Place one thumb above the other, just below the toes, and draw them out to each side of the foot. Release before repeating the stroke. Slowly move down the foot and back up to the starting position.

Gently squeeze and stretch the knuckles of each of the toes. Repeat all steps on the other foot.

Hold your partner's feet and take a few deep breaths together. Lie down with them to provide a comforting presence while they take the time to process their massage experience.

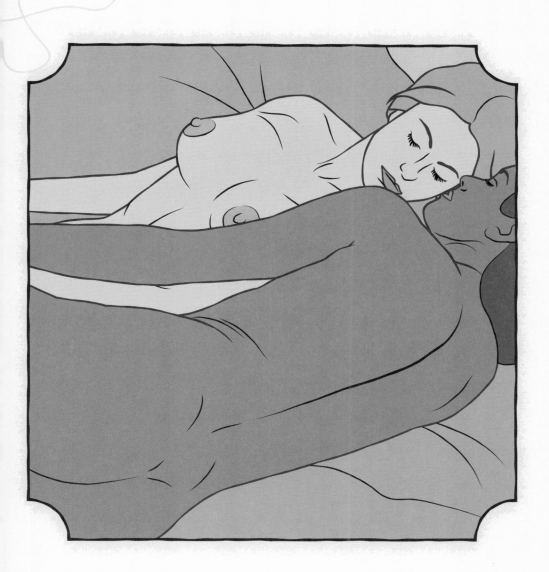

CLOSING YOUR PRACTICE

The importance of being present to one another extends to the afterglow period. Rest quietly together for as long as it takes for the receiver to come fully down from their experience. They may have emotions to process; be sleepy or full of energy; want to talk about the massage right away, or feel better keeping to themselves for a time. Just ride the wave, whatever it is. If you've agreed to switch roles directly after, reset your boundaries, intentions, and space (see page 66) when you're both ready.

Sharing your experience

After closing your practice, you and your partner may want to share your respective experiences. That is a great idea! Sharing favorite moments and ideas for future sessions is how you can build more personalized experiences. However, this isn't the time for the giver to seek validation and the receiver to dole out criticism, although this might be tempting. Instead, focus on what worked well for both of you, what you really enjoyed, what made you feel connected, relaxed, excited, etc. Of course, be honest about anything you'd like done differently, but be sure to offer constructive feedback and solutions that are relatively easy to attain. Consider keeping a small journal to record what you'd like to remember or change for future sessions. With open and kind communication, you can start to build your own shared pleasure map!

HELPFUL QUESTIONS

Use these questions to help process your massage
experience, as receiver or giver.

WHAT DID YOU MOST ENJOY FROM YOUR MASSAGE EXPERIENCE?
IDENTIFY AT LEAST THREE FAVORITE MOMENTS.

. . . .

MEDITATE ON THESE MOMENTS, HOW DOES
YOUR BODY FEEL WHEN YOU DO THAT?

. . . .

WHAT WOULD YOU LIKE TO DO DIFFERENTLY IN A FUTURE SESSION?

. . . .

HOW DID IT FEEL TO GIVE THE MASSAGE? DID YOU EXPERIENCE
ANY PLEASURE OF YOUR OWN WHILE GIVING?

. . . .

HOW DID IT FEEL TO RECEIVE THE MASSAGE? WAS IT CHALLENGING
OR EASY TO STAY FOCUSED ON YOUR SENSUAL EXPERIENCE?

LOVING YOURSELF ISN'T VANITY.
IT'S SANITY.

Katrina Mayer

CHAPTER 6

GOING SOLO

While much of this book is geared toward two people exchanging a sensual massage, it's important to know that all of these skills and techniques can be applied to you and your body alone. You can translate what you've learned to a solo self-pleasure session, including making boundaries, tuning into pleasure, learning your anatomy, and exploring sensation toys and tools.

I hope you take a few of these suggestions with you into your self-pleasure and see what happens! You are full of surprises waiting to be discovered. Happy trails!

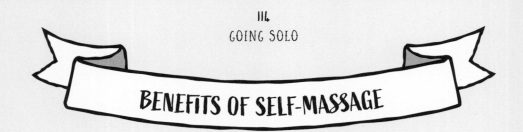

BENEFITS OF SELF-MASSAGE

It might start out feeling awkward or less exciting than spending time with a partner, but being with yourself in a curious, exploratory, and sensual way can become a profound self-care practice. Here is a sampling of the many benefits of self-massage.

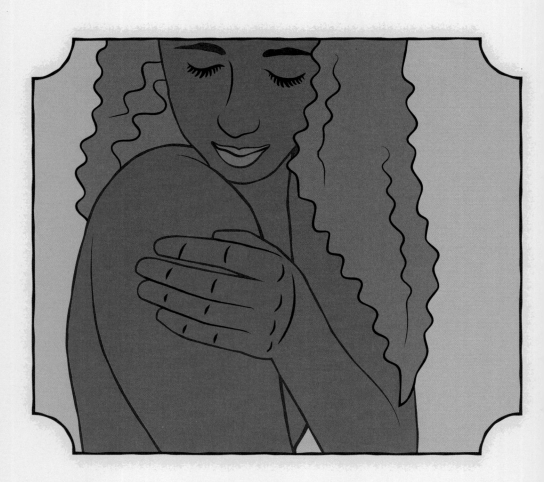

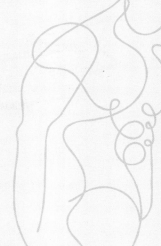

Meet the real you

Genuinely experiencing your body is a foundational step to having a realistic sense of self. The habit of projecting unrealistic ideals and expectations on our bodies comes with the territory of living in a body- (and sex-) negative culture. Spending time with the sensory reality of your body can help you befriend and find beauty, pleasure, and fun in what *is*.

Increase your self-love

Mindful self-touch boosts the production of serotonin, the feel-good hormone responsible for the warm and fuzzy feelings associated with intimacy, connection, relaxation, and contentment. You can give yourself a dose of that whenever you need!

Sharing is caring

Exploring yourself in this way provides valuable information that you can later share with a partner, if you wish, expanding your options for mutual pleasure. (You are, of course, more than welcome to keep your me-time private, a special experience that is just for you.)

Practice your boundaries

It is possible to become aware of your boundaries when you are alone. Giving yourself these moments of consent and choice is an excellent way to strengthen your boundaries, making them easier to communicate to others.

Practice being selfish: because it's all for you!

There is no one but yourself to please, get curious about, revel in, and marvel at. This is a space where being selfish is not only good but *required*.

SELF-MASSAGE TO EXPLORE BOUNDARIES

Exploring boundaries solo is a great foundation to build on with others. Unfortunately, even when we're by ourselves it's easy to ignore limits and bypass needs in order to get something "right," to hurry up, or to look a certain way, etc.

If this sounds familiar, consider self-massage time as an opportunity to address some of these habits. Try these exercises and notice any sensations or thoughts that come up for you:

CLAIMING YOURSELF

I learned this exercise from the inimitable Kimberly Ann Johnson, an author, teacher, sexological bodyworker, and mom.

TRY THIS

SIT OR LIE DOWN IN A PRIVATE, QUIET PLACE. BEGIN BY GENTLY PLACING YOUR HANDS ON THE **TOP OF YOUR HEAD**, FEELING THE CONTOURS OF YOUR SKULL UNDERNEATH. SAY TO YOURSELF, OUT LOUD IF POSSIBLE, "THIS IS MY HEAD."

REPEAT THIS PROCESS FOR **EVERY AREA** OF YOUR **BODY** THAT YOUR HANDS CAN REACH, TAKING SPECIAL CARE TO INCLUDE YOUR CHEST, BELLY, AND GENITALS. THESE ARE AREAS THAT CAN, AT TIMES, FEEL LIKE THEY BELONG TO SOMEONE OR SOMETHING ELSE: YOUR PARTNER, YOUR DOCTOR, YOUR CHILDREN, SOCIETAL STANDARDS, CULTURAL TABOOS, ETC. HOLD YOURSELF IN YOUR HANDS AND **CLAIM WHAT YOU TOUCH.** IT IS YOURS AND YOURS ALONE.

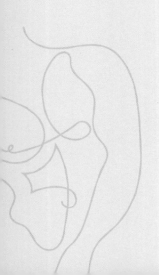

SELF-MASSAGE TO EXPLORE BOUNDARIES

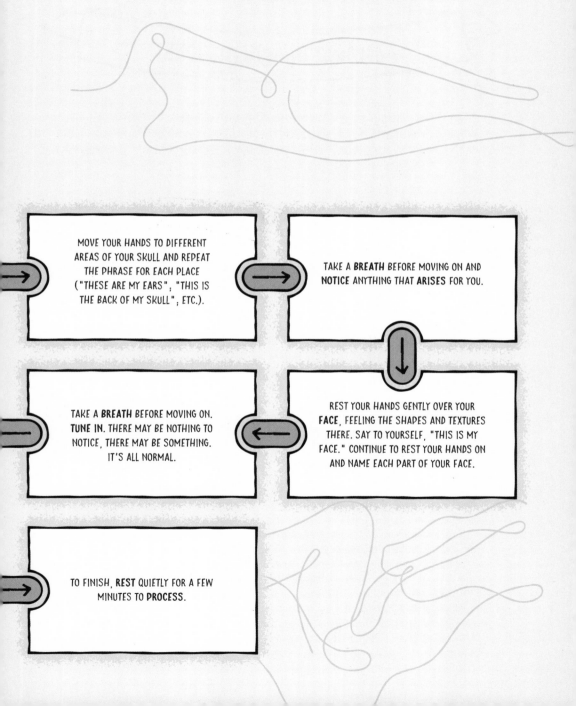

MOVE YOUR HANDS TO DIFFERENT AREAS OF YOUR SKULL AND REPEAT THE PHRASE FOR EACH PLACE ("THESE ARE MY EARS"; "THIS IS THE BACK OF MY SKULL"; ETC.).

TAKE A **BREATH** BEFORE MOVING ON AND **NOTICE** ANYTHING THAT **ARISES** FOR YOU.

TAKE A **BREATH** BEFORE MOVING ON. **TUNE IN.** THERE MAY BE NOTHING TO NOTICE, THERE MAY BE SOMETHING. IT'S ALL NORMAL.

REST YOUR HANDS GENTLY OVER YOUR **FACE**, FEELING THE SHAPES AND TEXTURES THERE. SAY TO YOURSELF, "THIS IS MY FACE." CONTINUE TO REST YOUR HANDS ON AND NAME EACH PART OF YOUR FACE.

TO FINISH, **REST** QUIETLY FOR A FEW MINUTES TO **PROCESS**.

EMBRACING GOLDILOCKS

While she's not always remembered fondly for her behavior in the home of the three bears, I like to think there's an alternative moral to the story of Goldilocks; that it's possible to get something "just right," and discovering that for yourself is time well spent.

We'll be applying this idea to touching ourselves, but it can be expanded to include any of the senses.

TRY THIS

TAKE A MOMENT TO **TUNE INTO** YOUR BODY, BREATHE EASILY AND **NOTICE** ANY **SENSATIONS**. ASK YOURSELF **WHERE YOU** WOULD **LIKE TO BE TOUCHED**. AND SEE IF AN ANSWER ARISES ON ITS OWN.

TRY THIS WITH A FEW DIFFERENT AREAS OF YOUR BODY AND SEE IF THE LEVELS OF PRESSURE AND YOUR SENSORY REACTIONS CHANGE. KEEP TUNING INTO YOUR BODY'S REACTIONS.

SAFETY AND LISTENING

These are only a few ways to explore your physical boundaries, but feel free to creatively experiment in your own way. You could place a circle of pillows around yourself when you self-massage, marking your specific and safe space. Even something as simple as locking the door to your room can go a long way to signaling safety to your system.

Throughout your practice, take a moment before diving into a physically sensitive or emotionally charged area of your body; ask yourself, do I want to be touched here? There is an answer waiting for you, however softly it may be spoken. It can be joyful to receive an enthusiastic "yes!" from your body, but sometimes it may say "no," and that's alright, too. Practice receiving any answer with gratitude and compassion.

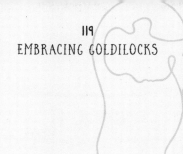

ONCE YOU'VE IDENTIFIED AN AREA THAT WANTS TOUCH, PLACE A HAND THERE. BEGIN WITH A **VERY LIGHT TOUCH** THAT FEELS LIKE IT'S **"NOT ENOUGH."** IT LEADS YOU TO WANTING MORE. ASK YOURSELF, HOW DO I KNOW I WANT MORE PRESSURE? WHERE DOES THAT COME FROM?

SLOWLY BEGIN TO **ADD MORE PRESSURE** UNTIL YOU REACH A PLACE WHERE IT FEELS **"JUST RIGHT"** TO THIS PART OF YOUR BODY. HOW DO YOU KNOW IT FEELS EXACTLY RIGHT? DOES THAT KNOWLEDGE HAVE A LOCATION OR SENSATION?

REVERSE FROM "TOO MUCH" TO "JUST RIGHT" AND FINALLY BACK TO "NOT ENOUGH," OBSERVING ANY CHANGES IN THE REST OF YOUR BODY.

KEEP **ADDING PRESSURE**, PASSING THE "JUST RIGHT" PLACE AND MOVING INTO **"TOO MUCH"** FOR A MOMENT. HOW DO YOU KNOW IT FEELS LIKE TOO MUCH PRESSURE? WHAT IN YOUR BODY LETS YOU KNOW THIS?

TIME WELL SPENT

Gradually, you can increase the amount of time you spend in the realms of "not enough" and "too much" (safely, of course). This begins to train your mind and body to notice more sensations outside of the normal way we touch ourselves, which can increase our capacity for new and different pleasures.

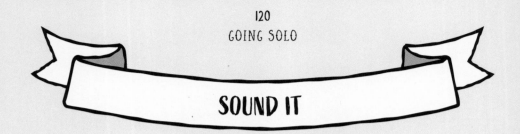

SOUND IT

Many of us learn to explore our sensuality and sexuality in total silence, for fear of being overheard or feeling ashamed of our behavior. Alternatively, we've been conditioned to mimic sounds we've learned are acceptable, whether through pornography, television, movies, or the judgment of partners.

This muzzling of our authentic voices has the unintended consequence of creating physical tension in the pelvis and the body in general, which decreases pleasurable sensations.

Making sound impacts the pelvis via your amazing vagus nerve, the tenth cranial nerve, which exits your spinal cord at the level of your ears. Along with myriad fascial and visceral connections, the vagus nerve forms a sensory highway between your throat, jaw, and pelvis, and the vibrations of your voice can directly stimulate this pathway. Tamping down the expressions of your voice can create tension in your jaw and throat, which then becomes mirrored in the pelvis. Freely making sounds creates vibrations that travel through your vagus nerve, fascia, and viscera down to your pelvic bowl, helping the musculature relax and expand. An additional benefit of this stimulation comes from the fact that the vagus nerve plays a large role in regulating your parasympathetic nervous system, the branch responsible for the rest-and-digest/tend-and-befriend drives that increase our ability to connect intimately with ourselves and others.

TRY THIS

Here are a few suggestions to incorporate sound into your self-pleasure:

PLAY YOUR FAVORITE MOOD MUSIC AND SING OR HUM ALONG. SERENADE YOURSELF!

INCLUDE AN AUDIBLE, OPEN-MOUTHED SIGH ON EVERY EXHALE. A LONG, DELICIOUS AAAAAH CAN GO FAR IN RELAXING YOUR BODY AND TURNING ON YOUR PARASYMPATHETIC NERVOUS SYSTEM. OVER TIME, THIS SIGH CAN BECOME WHATEVER SOUND YOU FEEL LIKE MAKING IN THE MOMENT.

WHEN YOU EXPERIENCE PLEASURE, SEE IF IT HAS A SOUND THAT YOU CAN MAKE WITH YOUR VOICE. IT COULD BE ANY SOUND: A GROWL, GROAN, SHOUT, LAUGH. LET IT TAKE YOU BY SURPRISE! THERE'S NO RIGHT OR WRONG HERE. SEE IF YOUR PLEASURE INCREASES OR CHANGES AS YOU EXPRESS IT IN THIS NEW WAY.

IF YOU ARE BUILDING AROUSAL, SEE IF YOU CAN RELAX YOUR JAW, TONGUE, AND THROAT. NOTICE ANY CHANGES IN YOUR AROUSAL OR THE SENSATIONS IN AND AROUND YOUR PELVIS WHEN YOU DO.

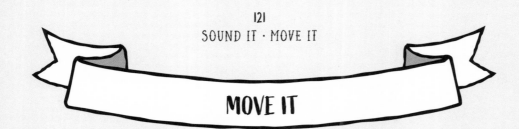

MOVE IT

How often do you change positions in your typical self-pleasure practice? Have you ever tried it standing up? Walking around? Dancing? All of these are possible ideas for bringing more moves to your me-time.

Movement changes your energy levels and can shift your state fairly quickly. For example, stand up right now and shake your whole body for a full three minutes, then see how you feel. Maybe you're brighter, full of tingles, and more energized; that's just one example of how movement can change your sensations.

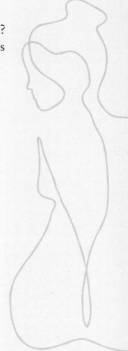

TRY THIS

Try these exercises to get moving in your practice:

PLAY WITH GOING BACK AND FORTH BETWEEN MOVEMENT AND STILLNESS. WHAT HAPPENS TO YOUR ENERGY IN THESE DIFFERENT STATES?

SET A TIMER FOR FIVE MINUTES WHEN YOU PRACTICE. EACH TIME THE TIMER GOES OFF, SWITCH YOUR POSITION. HOW DO YOUR SENSATIONS DIFFER FROM ONE POSITION TO THE NEXT?

DANCE IT OUT! PUT ON A PLAYLIST THAT PUTS YOU IN THE MOOD AND SELF-PLEASURE WHILE DANCING. WHAT DOES YOUR PLEASURE LOOK LIKE IN A DANCE? HOW WOULD YOU EXPRESS IT WITH YOUR WHOLE BODY?

TOUCH IT

Solo self-pleasure is a perfect place to observe our habits around touch. Understandably, many of us stick with the tried-and-true methods that get us to where we'd like to go, be that to orgasm or elsewhere. There's nothing wrong with that!

I'm not here to suggest you throw the baby out with the bath water, but it's worth it to learn how to switch it up. Your whole body is an amazing organ of perception with innumerable roads to pleasure. Why not use your hands to travel down some new roads?

Expanding your capacity for pleasure

Anytime we change a familiar routine or try something for the first time it can feel strange, even awkward. If you are trying to build arousal, you may find these new strategies affect that climb in the beginning, bringing it down or sometimes stopping it. That's normal, and part of the process of expanding your capacity for pleasure. Look at it like an experiment, open-ended and with no agenda. Then, whenever you want, you can return to the more familiar ways of being with your body. You may find that these are enriched by your experimentation. In the end, I hope that these tools bring you a deeper knowledge of yourself, your pleasures, and your body.

TRY THIS

TUNE INTO YOUR BODY AND SEE IF THERE'S ANY AREA THAT WANTS **TOUCH**. BEGIN TOUCHING THIS PLACE IN YOUR USUAL WAY, THE TOUCH YOU'RE **FAMILIAR** WITH AND KNOW BRINGS YOU PLEASURE.

TRY THIS FOR AT LEAST **20 MINUTES**, SWITCHING YOUR TOUCH EVERY FIVE SO YOU EXPLORE AT LEAST **FOUR** DIFFERENT **VARIATIONS**. KEEP TRACK OF WHAT YOU LIKE AND DISLIKE.

CURIOSITY

The tools given on pages 120–123 can help you explore new ways to be with your body, shift habits, and imbue your self-touch with a sense of curiosity and playfulness. I give all credit to Joseph Kramer, the man who created Sexological Bodywork, for originally gathering these easy and practical ways to bring mindfulness to a self-pleasure practice.

SET A TIMER FOR **FIVE MINUTES** AND WHEN IT GOES OFF SWITCH UP YOUR TOUCH BY TRYING SOMETHING THAT FEELS NOVEL AND **OUTSIDE** OF YOUR **USUAL ROUTINE**. CONSIDER THE SENSUAL TOUCH TECHNIQUES DETAILED ON PAGES 58–61. IS THERE ONE THAT IS LESS FAMILIAR TO YOU? TRY IT ON YOURSELF.

WHEN YOU SWITCH YOUR TOUCH, WHAT DO YOU **NOTICE** IN YOUR **BODY**? WHEN YOU FIND A TOUCH YOU LIKE, HOW DOES THAT INFORMATION COME FROM YOUR BODY? WHAT ABOUT WHEN YOU FIND A TOUCH YOU DON'T LIKE?

AFTER ANOTHER FIVE MINUTES, **SWITCH AGAIN**. HAVE YOU TRIED IMPACT YET? OR SCRATCHING? TAPPING? SQUEEZING? JIGGLING? JUST HAVE FUN AND EXPLORE.

KNOW YOUR ROUTINE

If, or when, you touch an erogenous zone of your body during your self-pleasure practice, observe your normal routine. How do you typically touch yourself and what does that feel like? What reactions does it create in your body? Getting clear on our usual self-touch routines helps us to recognize patterns and gives us more choice about when and how to alter them.

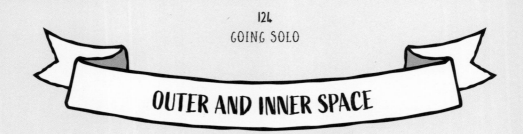

OUTER AND INNER SPACE

When you're by yourself, it may not seem so important to set up the space like you would with another person. I believe this is a missed opportunity, however. Creating a pleasant environment for yourself can enhance the experience by stimulating your senses, increasing relaxation, and reminding yourself that this is a special occasion, separate from your everyday routines and responsibilities.

External space

Consider the space around you. Does it need to be tidied up? Does clutter distract you? Just do the basics to clear it up; there's no need to deep clean each time you want to set aside some time for yourself. Can you adjust the lights, temperature, or the decor to your liking? What colors, scents, sounds, and textures most relax and please you? Just a few of these can make the difference between a room that feels uninteresting to one that feels inviting.

Internal space

Once you've considered your external environment, turn your attention to your internal environment. Just as you would with a partner, take some time to clarify what intentions you have for your practice. What are you interested in experiencing, or curious to learn about yourself?

An intention is different from a goal—you don't arrive at an intention, but it informs the steps you take. Maybe you will end up in surprising new territory, guided as you are by any number of intentions: to try a new pleasure tool, to access more self-love, to explore the eroticism of a certain part of your body. Once again, curiosity and open-mindedness are the keys to unlocking new doors to pleasure, self-awareness, and play.

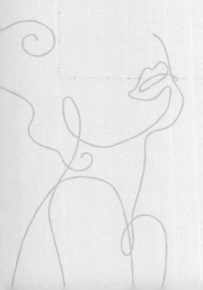

HELPFUL QUESTIONS

These questions may help you to understand and
improve your self-massage experiences.

HOW DO YOU NORMALLY SELF-PLEASURE? WHAT DO YOU LIKE ABOUT IT?
WHAT, IF ANYTHING, WOULD YOU LIKE TO SHIFT OR CHANGE?

....

WHICH OF THE PLEASURE TOOLS DO YOU THINK WOULD BE EASY TO
INCORPORATE? WHICH DO YOU THINK WOULD BE CHALLENGING TO USE?

....

HOW DO YOU KNOW WHEN YOU'VE DISCOVERED SOMETHING YOU REALLY
ENJOY? OR WHEN YOU DISCOVER SOMETHING YOU DISLIKE? WHERE
DOES THIS INFORMATION LIVE IN YOUR BODY?

....

HOW CAN YOU SET UP YOUR SPACE TO MAKE IT
MOST INVITING AND SENSUAL FOR YOURSELF?

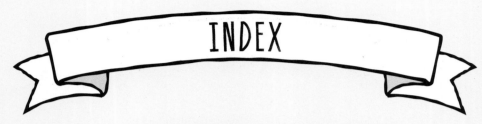

INDEX

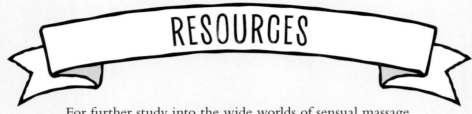

RESOURCES

For further study into the wide worlds of sensual massage, boundaries, erotic education, human anatomy, and more, these resources should serve you well.

Anatomy

Jack Morin, Ph. D. *Anal Pleasure and Health*

R. Louis Schultz, Ph. D., *Out in the Open: The Complete Male Pelvis*

Sheri Winston, CNM, RN, BSN, LMT, *Women's Anatomy of Arousal: Secret Maps to Buried Pleasure*

Boundaries

Betty Martin, teacher and developer of The Wheel of Consent: *bettymartin.org* The School of Consent: *schoolofconsent.org*

Erotic massage

Caffyn Jesse's books and free resources: *erospirit.ca*

Joseph Kramer, the founder of Sexological Bodywork, has two websites dedicated to solo and partner practices: *orgasmicyoga.com* and *eroticmassage.com*

Intersex, non-binary, and transgender information

Gender Spectrum: *genderspectrum.org*

GLAAD's resources for trans youth and adults: *glaad.org/transgender/resources*

Interact Advocates for Intersex Youth: *interactadvocates.org*

Intersex Society of North America: *isna.org*

Pelvic bodywork

Ellen Heed: *ellenheed.com*

Kimberly Ann Johnson: *magamama.com*

Tami Lynn Kent, developer of Holistic Pelvic Care: *wildfeminine.com*

Pamela Samuelson: *embodyworkla.com*

Sexological bodywork

Association of Certified Sexological Bodyworkers: *sexologicalbodyworkers.org*

Institute of Somatic Sexology: *instituteofsomaticsexology.com*

ACKNOWLEDGMENTS
I would like to thank Joseph Kramer, the founder of sexological bodywork, and Deej Juventin and Uma Ayelet-Furman, my wonderful teachers. I am eternally grateful to Pamela Samuelson and Kimberly Ann Johnson, the first sexological bodyworkers I had the privilege of working with and who inspired me to pursue this training. Many thanks, also, to Betty Martin who generously let me use pieces of her work with The Wheel of Consent to create the chapter on boundaries and consent. Big hugs and kisses to Ondra, Matt, and Pam for exploring ideas with me, proofreading, and being so supportive.